The Daylight Diet

Divine Eating for Superior Health and Digestion

Paul Nison

Disclaimer

The information presented herein represents the view of the author as of the date of publication. Every effort has been made to make this book as accurate as possible. It was written with the intention of providing information about eating a Daylight Diet for superior health and digestion.

This book is not intended as medical advice. All information contained herein is not intended as a diagnosis, cure, or treatment for any disease or ailment. Because the Daylight Diet changes one's diet and often produces an initial cleansing reaction, readers are advised to educate themselves adequately and seek advice from a qualified holistic or medical professional when needed. In addition, the author, publisher, and/or distributors of this book are not responsible for any adverse detoxification effects or consequences resulting from the use of any suggestions or procedures described herein.

Cover design and text layout: Enrique Candioti

Back cover photo: Durga Garcia

Published by:
343 Publishing Company
P.O. Box 16156
West Palm beach, FL 33416
www.Paulnison.com

Printed in Canada
ISBN # 978-0-9675286-5-6

WHAT OTHERS ARE SAYING

"With Paul's approach, you will cut down radically the number of hours you need to sleep and will wake fully energized after a night of beautiful and enjoyable dreams."

— Viktoras Kulvinskas, M.S. author and co-founder, of the world famous Hippocrates Health Institute, www.viktoraslive.org

"This important contribution highlights a critical aspect of biological health. Paul's easy-to-understand explanation about timing your food consumption is as crucial to employ as the choices themselves. Be well!"

— Drs. Anna Maria and Brian Clement, PhD, LN, authors, Directors of Hippocrates Health Institute, www.Hippocratesinst.org

"For more than 30 years, I have dealt with cancer patients who could have all profited massively from Paul Nison's books and knowledge. Paul is his own best model: He walks his talk and lives what he teaches. His new book, *The Daylight Diet*, is a new breakthrough in Paul's work. He demonstrates for everybody how easy it can be to live a healthier, happier, and more energetic life. I will make this book a must-read for everybody I care for. Paul Nison's insight and experience give the reader a new way to understand and achieve better health, energy, and quality of life.

— Dr. Leonard Coldwell, NMD PHD DNM CNHP, author of *Instinct Based Medicine: How to survive your illness and your doctor* www.Instinctbasedmedicine.com

"I've read many books about health in the last 60 years. *The Daylight Diet* by Paul Nison is one of the best books that I've ever read, with a very important, profound message— that is often overlooked—as he expounds on the wisdom of eating during daylight hours. For those who are not willing to settle for mediocrity and want to strive to be the most they can, this book is a must read."

— Dr. Fred Bisci, PhD, nutritionist, author of *Your Healthy Journey* www.Fredbisci4health.com

"Paul Nison's book, *The Daylight Diet*, tells about the nightmares of eating late at night. This goes right along with the message I have been teaching all my life. Our digestion has its highest absorption when the sun is at the highest point in the sky. We should wake at dawn, and sleep after sunset. I can truly say, even at my age of 86 years, that I have benefited from Paul's insights and especially this important message in his latest book."

— **Jay Kordich, author of *The Father of Juicing* www.Juicedaddy.com**

"A key to my longevity is that I eat the same time every day and never eat at nighttime."

— **Bernando LaPallo, 108 years old, author of *Ageless Live More*, www.Agelesslivemorestore.com**

"Paul Nison's book ought to be required reading for anyone seeking to embrace the full value of a calorie-restricted, raw foods regimen. I endorse Paul's *Daylight Diet* because it's very similar to my own Quantum Eating plan.

— **Tonya Zavasta, author of *Your Right to Be Beautiful: Miracle of Raw Foods* and *Quantum Eating: The Ultimate Rejuvenation*, www.Beautifulonraw.com**

"*The Daylight Diet* is an informative guide to eating in harmony with the very cycle of life. Gleaned from extensive study of the habits of the world's healthiest people, the eating plan outlined by Paul Nison can add years to your life and life to your years."

— **Jordan Rubin, NMD, PhD, author and Founder of Garden of Life, www.JordanRubin.com**

"In my research over the last 40 years, I have found that nighttime eating is counterproductive and best avoided. Eating at the ideal time for digestion during the day and foregoing eating at nighttime has proven to be enormously beneficial for many people. Paul has very skillfully covered this subject with clarity and thoroughness in his excellent new book, *The Daylight Diet.*"

— **Harvey Diamond, author, www.harveydiamond.com**

DEDICATION

This book is dedicated to Dr. Dio Lewis, who preached about eating a Daylight Diet in the 1800s and had a passion for teaching temperance in all things. Finding his books was a blessing, and it gives me great pleasure to share his lifelong work with the readers of *The Daylight Diet.*

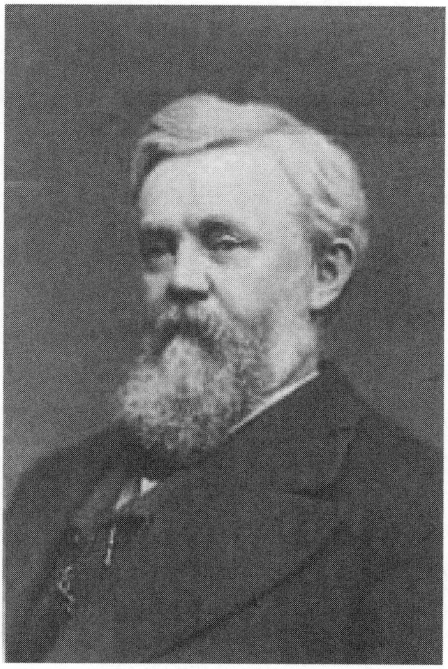

ACKNOWLEDGMENTS

Many people helped me with this book. I want to thank everyone but can only name a few. Special thanks to Yahweh, Our Creator, for blessing me with the knowledge and wisdom to understand His divine time schedule; to Tonya Zavasta, Fred Bisci, Stanley Bass, Jay Kordich, Harvey Diamond and Jordan Rubin, for your knowledge and history to Doug Mitchell, for teaching me about the daily times of Yahweh; and to Bernando LaPallo, who proves, at 108 years young, that the Daylight Diet works!

Thanks to all the people who helped proofread and transform my ideas into this book, especially Carol Wiley Lorente, Hope Richards, Heather Wolcott, Alvin Last, Megan Orr, Bob Avery, Jeanie Rosenthal, Joel Brody, Bharata and Enrique Candioti.

An extra thanks to Nikki Jones and my friends at Health Research Books for reprinting Dr. Lewis's book *Talks about People's Stomachs,* which I often quote herein. If you would like to purchase a copy, please visit my website at www.rawlife.com.

And most importantly, thank you to my beautiful wife and daughter, Andrea and Noa Raquel Nison.

CONTENTS

Foreword xiii
Introduction 15

Part 1: The History of Eating 25

Chapter 1
Good Digestion, Good Health 27
Less is always more where good food is concerned

Chapter 2
Late-Night Eating 39
Just say no to eating after sunset

Chapter 3
Daylight Diet by Design 45
Break with custom, and be healthy

Chapter 4
The Health Writers Hall of Fame 57
Good ideas gone wrong

Chapter 5
Breaking the Nightly Fast 79
What you need to know about breakfast

Chapter 6
Quality and Quantity 83
Late-night eating has got to go

Part 2: Digestion and the Daylight Diet 89

Chapter 7
Let the Sun Shine 91
It's sunlight that really gets digestion moving

Chapter 8
No More Bedtime Snacks 99
The importance of rest and sleep to digestion

Chapter 9
Two Meals a Day 115
Everything you think you know about eating is wrong

Chapter 10
Adrenal Fatigue **131**
How TV, sugar, caffeine, and computers are making you sick

Part 3: Preparing Yourself to Eat Less Food, Less Often 139

Chapter 11
Understanding Nighttime Hunger **141**
Maybe we need better food

Chapter 12
Learning to Adapt **147**
Change in the right direction

Chapter 13
The Power of Temperance **151**
The essence of the Daylight Diet

Chapter 14
Endurance and Enthusiasm **157**
It's all in the planning

Chapter 15
The Formula for Health **161**
Good digestion equals good health

Chapter 16
The Daily Detox **167**
A clean body needs less food

Chapter 17
Emotions, Environment, and Social Changes **175**
Dealing with your friends, your family, and yourself

Part 4: Achieving The Daylight Diet 191

Chapter 18
Take Time to Schedule. **193**
Planning is crucial for success

Chapter 19
The Daylight Diet Program **199**
The three stages to health

Chapter 20
Monitoring Your Health 207
How to tell if you're really healthy

Chapter 21
Good Counsel 215
Whom to turn to

Chapter 22
Exceptional Circumstances 219
Is the Daylight Diet ever a bad idea?

Chapter 23
Putting It All Together 223
There's more to it than just food

Conclusion 227
Time to take action

A Final Thought 231
The wonderful mind of Dr. Dio Lewis

Recipes 235

Nut Milks 235
Salads and Salad Dressings 236
Dips, Spreads, and Sauces 240
Blended Meals 242
About the Author 245
Resources 247
Other Books by Paul Nison 249
Bibliography 251
Index 255

FOREWORD

James Watson, the co-discoverer of DNA in 1953, said on the 50th anniversary of his discovery, "*In 50 years, we will have drugs that will let us eat as much as we want without gaining weight.*" Dr. Watson might be right—who knows? But think about it: what an astonishing proposition to have as a goal, to eat as much as we want.

That proposition certainly has curb appeal in our culture of eat, eat, and eat. And here comes *The Daylight Diet*, in which Paul Nison says: Eat less. Eat only during the daytime. Eat raw. In this, Paul has my heartiest concurrence.

The health of people who follow a carefully crafted raw foods lifestyle seem to set them apart—not above ordinary humanity, but as a standard of what human beings can achieve. When we're with such people, we come away wishing that we knew the secret of their glowing health. Paul is one of these people.

In *The Daylight Diet*, Paul shows that the two-meals-a-day plan is neither new nor radical. His historical examples show we have a wealth of good role models for our "modern" nutritional plan. His detailed research gives us a valuable mode of defense against outsiders who become hysterical about our not getting enough nutrients like essential fatty acids, proteins, and so on—you know the drill.

I've been following a two-meals-a-day plan for several years now. I've discovered this is the best anti-aging and beautifying tool there is. In my early fifties, I've been able to turn back the clock and look and feel better than ever.

Paul Nison's Daylight Diet teaches how to make a smooth transition to eating less and, not eating late at night. If I can do it day after day, you, using this book as a guide, also can embrace *the Daylight Diet*.

Advocating "less eating" will remain an unpopular theme at least for the near future. In a culture of excess, eating less—like any kind of temperance—feels like a deprivation, feels hard. But when you combine low-calorie eating with eating raw, you'll in fact reach an ideal combination that will actually make your life *easier*.

I hope this book by Paul Nison has found you, that special person who is ready for his message, ready to break free from imposed cultural beliefs, ready to reap amazing health and anti-aging benefits. Follow Paul's advice, and you'll be rewarded with a profound transformation not only in body, but in mind, in your outlook on life, and in your consciousness. You will become, in effect, whatever your chronological age, a young adult—and *better* than what you once were.

— Tonya Zavasta, author of *Your Right to Be Beautiful: Miracle of Raw Foods* and *Quantum Eating: The Ultimate Rejuvenation* www. Beautifulonraw.com

INTRODUCTION

The raw food diet revolution is part of a health movement that started long before I was born, and I am blessed to be an active and vocal part of it. I have dedicated my entire adult life to promoting a diet that emphasizes raw food, not only because it is the most healthful way to eat, but also because it gave me my health back, and, by doing so, it gave me my life back. And when that happened, it provided an important way for me to help people.

Almost 10 years have passed since I published my first book, *The Raw Life*; it has inspired many people to give the raw food diet a try. People often send me messages thanking me for *The Raw Life* and telling me how much it convinced them to "go raw." It is very encouraging to know my book has helped change so many people's lives, and, I believe, helped save a few as well.

The raw food movement is flourishing. More people are writing books about eating raw foods; people are sharing their stories on the Internet about how the raw food diet has helped them, and restaurants continue to add more raw food options to their menus.

As healthful as the raw food diet is, it's not all it can be. Since I've become involved in the raw food movement, I've noticed a problem that continues to worsen as the diet's popularity grows: Some people who have adopted the raw food lifestyle are confused about the best way to go about it, and there is division and disagreement about the best way to implement the diet for the utmost health. Some people in the movement are promoting raw food diets that are high in fruit; others say eating a lot of fruit isn't a good thing. Then there are the people who argue the pros and cons of high fat versus low fat.

Splits within the health movement are nothing new. Health writers have always disagreed about which remedies are truly helpful and which ones aren't. Besides, things aren't always as they appear. When I first came to the raw food movement, the diet appeared so straightforward to me: eat high-quality, uncooked fruits, vegetables, nuts, and seeds. I couldn't have imagined that people would have such different views about eating so simply. Obviously, not all raw diets were the same. As I continued on my journey to health, I accepted that there were going to be differences within the raw movement, and that I would have to find what worked best.

When I first started teaching the raw food diet, my message was simple: Eat raw fruits, vegetables, nuts, and seeds, as much as you want, anytime you want. As long as the food is raw, you will be fine. I've learned a great deal over the years and now have a very different outlook.

I have learned to keep an open mind, and, as I continue to grow, my message continues to evolve as I discover what works and what doesn't. As a result, I've discovered some key components to healthful eating that I think many health teachers today are missing. These key components are the basis of this book.

It is common knowledge that the quality of our food is vital to superior health. Eating fruits and vegetables raw, ripe, fresh, and organic is the ideal in terms of quality. However, an extremely important point often not discussed is that it's not only the quality of our food that matters, but also how we eat and when we eat. It's bewildering that, even with this unbelievably simple information I reveal and teach in this book, people will still refuse to change their eating habits. The fact is, they will never achieve the highest level of health on a raw food diet if they do it the way many teachers today are suggesting. (Even more disturbing is that these people make idols out of the teachers who teach these misleading messages.)

Where has all this division left us? Some people eating a raw food diet will see improvements in their health, but, after a few years, the majority of them will be sicker than when they started. Their conditions will worsen because they seem to be more addicted to a concept than to the truth, and, as a result, they will be more confused about what is truly healthful.

The Bible as textbook

I have always had a strong desire to help people, and that desire intensified after years of suffering with inflammatory bowel disease (IBD). It's exactly what the name states: inflammation of the bowel (colon). The doctors didn't have a cure then, and, to this day, they are still searching for one. I discovered the cure from reading and studying. After years of pain and suffering, I was shocked to discover the actual cause of my illness was my unhealthful diet and lifestyle. When I changed my diet, I began to see light at the end of a very dark tunnel, and I told myself that, when I made it out of that darkness, I was going to dedicate the rest of my life to helping those who suffer with diseases caused by their diets.

My passion and desire to help people has brought me to where I am today—a full-time teacher and health writer—and led me to write this book you hold in your hand. During my amazing path to healing, I learned about the connection between health and digestion: The better our digestion, the better our health. Many books I studied spoke about this connection, so it really wasn't a revelation, but the books didn't talk about how to fully obtain ultimate digestion. That is the revelation I had, and that I'm going to explain in this book.

Where did this revelation of mine originate? One of the most incredible health teachers I have ever met, and who is now a great friend, is nutritionist Dr. Fred Bisci. Dr. Bisci is more knowledgeable about health than anyone I have ever known. When I first met him, I asked him how he knew so much and where he learned it all. He told me no books teach what he learned, and that there is only one place to get the knowledge he had.

I was at the edge of my seat as I waited for him to tell me where the place was. I never expected what I was about to hear. Dr. Bisci told me he was a Christian and had a personal relationship with God. He said he asked God to bless him with an understanding about the human body, health, and healing. Without a doubt, his prayers were answered: I have never met anyone who knows more on the topic, and anyone who spends any time with him will agree. But I was not ready to hear that God gave him the knowledge; I wanted to find the information and study it for myself.

At the time, I didn't have a personal relationship with God. I had mixed opinions and ideas about God. I certainly believed in a Higher Power, but I was determined to learn about diet and healing from health books written by experts, not from God. It turned out that I did learn about health from books, but I was way off the mark in my prediction that I would be unable to learn more about health through a relationship with God.

Years after meeting Fred Bisci, and after some remarkable circumstances, I became interested in reading the Bible for the first time in my life. At first, it was only to see what the Bible had to say about health. Someone at a lecture I presented had said there was information about diet and health in the Bible, and this sparked my interest. It wasn't too long before I developed a special personal relationship with God and accepted Yeshua (Jesus) as my Savior. The Bible became the best health book I ever read. I began to pray for wisdom, and I asked God to use me to help people, to show me what people were missing, and to reveal it to them in a way where they too would see the light. Eventually, I received the revelation about the Daylight Diet.

My revelation

While researching my last book, *The Formula for Health*, I learned that what motivates most people to change their diet is:

1. To cure an existing illness
2. To avoid getting an illness
3. To stay looking young and to have more energy.

In *The Formula for Health*, I focused on the first two factors in the list and discussed how to heal and avoid disease. The ideas in this book you have in your hands will certainly help you achieve those goals as well, but its main focus is on the third factor in the list: slowing down the aging process and enjoying an abundance of energy and good health.

After traveling to many countries (often more in a year than most people travel in a lifetime), I've seen many eating patterns. The majority of people seem to have one thing in common: They are addicted to eating in excess. Very few people I've met in my travels have been able to practice temperance while eating.

I understand gluttony well. For most of my life, prior to my revelation, I too was a glutton. However, unlike the majority, I became wiser, obedient, and disciplined. I stepped back from feeding that addiction. I remember Fred Bisci telling me a long time ago that one of the keys to eating healthfully was to eat very little and not focus on the temporary pleasure food brings. I'll never forget what he said: "When you find as much pleasure *not* eating as you do eating, you will have overcome the addiction."

I know some people who force themselves to eat less, and they are not happy: They miss the pleasure of eating too much. They would rather live with the pain from overindulgence than go without the temporary pleasure. But once you understand that eating less is better for your health, it makes consuming less more enjoyable.

I have experienced how stepping back makes it much easier to see the full picture. When you are caught in a daily routine of giving in to your addictions, your life becomes almost like a matrix. It becomes almost impossible for you to see what's really happening.

Practicing temperance in eating will rejuvenate your whole body and rid you of most health problems. Your goal should be to reduce the number of meals you consume and reduce the amount of food in those meals, while making sure you are consuming the highest quality food. The real key to success is to avoid eating at nighttime, and go to sleep on an empty stomach.

Food shouldn't be a daily struggle. I can attest that it may not be easy at first, but to be truly successful, you will have to change your thinking along with your diet.

Where to begin?

Without changing any food in your diet, just do this one thing: Don't eat late in the day. You will get better sleep, have better digestion, slow down the aging process, have more energy, and feel wonderful. Just stop eating late in the day—especially when it's dark outside—and experience for yourself the great results.

This may not be as simple as it sounds. Overindulgence of food is one of the most common addictions, and, in my experience, it's one of the hardest to break; eating at nighttime is even more addictive. Nighttime binge eating has become a common cause of obesity, sickness, and disease. There are even eating disorders called night-eating syndrome—eating mostly at night—and sleep-eating, when people actually eat while they're asleep without even knowing it.

In my lectures, I often tell people there is a difference between a habit and an addiction. A habit is something we enjoy doing on a regular basis, but when we find out it's not good for us, we can stop the behavior. Sometimes it takes a while, but with hard work, eventually the habit is broken. An addiction is something we enjoy doing on a regular basis, but when we discover it is not good for us, we make excuses to keep doing it. That's when we know it's an addiction and not a habit. We must change our food addictions into habits, and then break free from them.

Eating a raw diet means little for your health if you are going to overeat, eat at the wrong times, and eat unhealthful food. If you are drinking green smoothies all day and continuing to eat until late at night, or you're eating tons of bananas a day, or if most of your diet includes (raw) junk food, such as chocolate, dried fruit, and raw recipes, you shouldn't be so puzzled when you find you don't achieve your desired results.

The key to health from a dietary standpoint (from every standpoint, actually), is the consistent practice of temperance: Don't overeat. The quality of your food is important, but you are wasting your time if you are not allowing the natural capabilities of your body to utilize that food correctly. Your system can't stay healthy if it's being bombarded with too much food, too often, and late at night. Of course you are going to feel better if last week you were eating tons of McDonald's every day, and this week you are eating tons of produce instead, but you're still overeating, which, in the long run, will cause health issues.

The body is amazing. It can handle most junk food and processed food if they're eaten in very small amounts, but in larger amounts, many health problems result because the worse the food, the harder it is for the body to handle it. Yet, I have come to know that, even if you are eating high-quality food too often and at the wrong times, damage is still taking place. You may not notice it right away, but stressing the body's organs in any way adds to sickness and disease.

I've learned the hard way. When I started eating a raw diet, I ate and ate and ate. I ate more exotic fruits than anyone I know, and I also overate other fruits and so-called healthful recipes. With the knowledge and help I gained from Dr. Fred Bisci and classic health writers such as Arnold Ehret, I learned to stop overeating, and now I finally enjoy the health and energy that many people are searching for.

Relax and enjoy

On the television show "Bizarre Foods," host Andrew Zimmern travels the world, eating extremely gross foods that are common in different countries. When I first saw the show several years ago, I figured that either the show would be canceled, or the host would be dead very soon. The funny thing is that, although Andrew is a little overweight, he is still very much alive.

My point is this: The human body is amazing. Too many people today are getting stressed out by every tiny bit of food that crosses their lips. Yes, the quality of food you eat is important, but if the stress of trying to be healthy creates more harm than the foods you are trying to avoid, then your chosen diet and lifestyle may not be worth it. I laugh when I see raw foodists question whether the cashew they ate was truly raw or if the nori sheet was toasted. If 98 percent of the foods you are eating are raw, the other two percent isn't going to harm you. On the contrary, that two percent may just be what keeps you sane. Stop worrying so much, and enjoy your life and your food.

I spent many years stressing over the food I ate. I have finally come to the conclusion that we are all going to die someday no matter what we do. That does not justify treating our bodies badly or deliberately living in an unhealthful way; there are plenty of reasons for us to chill out and relax. If you eat a 100 percent raw food diet, great, but if it's too stressful, then eating a little cooked food is not going to kill you. If cooked food really killed us, we would all be dead. It is overeating any food, whether cooked or raw, that does us in.

I am a history buff. I love to study people who lived in the 1700s and 1800s - especially those who shared my passion for health, diet, and the Bible. It is interesting that, in all my research, I have never read about organizations raising money to combat diseases or marathons to raise money for researching new drugs to control disease in that era. What I have discovered is that people ate whole foods, practiced temperance while eating, and lived a simple life. Processed foods were not available like they are today, and big food companies weren't poisoning the soil to plant their crops.

Another thing that amazes me about the past is the difference in communication compared to today. While I'm reading about health in the 1800s, for example, I know the authors of those books had limited ability to see works by other authors, yet they come to the same conclusions: Eat frugally, and eat wholesome foods.

Make it happen

I am convinced you can throw away every diet and health book you own, as long as you follow my simple plan:

- Provide your body with the required nutrients, mostly from fresh, raw, organic fruits, vegetables, nuts, and seeds.
- Go to sleep on an empty stomach to provide your body time to digest your food and keep the colon clean.

To make that happen:

- Do not eat more than two or three times a day.
- No snacking in between meals.
- Wait at least four hours between meals.
- Do not eat within four hours of going to sleep for the night.
- Do not eat when it is dark outside

When you do eat:

- Do not consume processed foods.
- Do not eat while stressed.
- Chew your food well.

Our Creator designed our bodies so amazingly well. We need to enjoy living. This doesn't mean going out and eating anything you desire, but don't lock yourself in your house because you are too worried about temptation. Instead of worrying, become aware. Arrange your daily schedule efficiently so you can eat the proper amounts at the proper times. Control your appetite. Even more important than the food you eat is what you do with your time. Enjoy life!

PART 1

The History of Eating

CHAPTER 1

GOOD DIGESTION, GOOD HEALTH

Less is always more where good food is concerned.

The human body is amazing when we treat it the way we're supposed to.

We were designed to eat certain types of foods—raw, fresh, organic fruits, vegetables, nuts, and seeds—to keep our digestive systems moving and clean. It took me years to understand that good health comes only when we have good digestion, and that good digestion only results when we eat properly and healthfully.

As a teenager, I became interested in playing sports and began to pay close attention to what I ate. I wanted to be bigger and stronger, and I assumed eating more was the answer. It wasn't until I was diagnosed with inflammatory bowel disease (IBD) at age 20 that I discovered I had been eating a very unhealthful diet. Prior to my illness, I thought I looked fine and felt wonderful. My endurance and strength were superb. I ignored my growing belly, problem skin, and unpleasant attitude. Nothing was going to keep me from eating anything I wanted.

Reminiscing about my teenage years now that I am much more aware, I realize it wasn't endurance but *stimulation* that kept me going—stimulation from unhealthful, processed, chemically-laden foods. Countless children and teenagers appear to thrive on unhealthful food, but eventually the damage they are building will supersede the stimulation, resulting in a state of disease.

My worst health nightmare came with the diagnosis of IBD, also known as ulcerative colitis, and Crohn's disease. My condition brought about everything I was striving to avoid: I was exercising to be big and strong, and I became weaker and smaller; at one point, my weight plummeted to 118 pounds. (Talk about humbling experience). My main concern was how to avoid the symptoms of my illness, because I didn't want to look skinny. To a young man, a scrawny appearance is worse than the pain of illness. I've since overcome that shallow thinking, but, back then, I was young and naïve, so focused on looking good on the outside that I was not interested in dealing with the inside. Finding a cure was not my top priority: I urgently had to stop the weight loss that came with IBD.

In addition, I had to reverse the muscle loss that resulted from malnutrition: Even though I was eating, and eating a lot, I was not able to completely assimilate nutrients because the disease prevented my colon from doing one of its main jobs: metabolizing nutrients from food. My solution was to eat more, and to eat more calorie-dense meals. High-fat and high-protein foods became the mainstay of my diet, but the more I ate, the worse my condition seemed to get.

Give it up.

After years of hospital visits and trying drug after drug with no improvement, I decided I would just give up. This came on a day when I was in my bathroom, the toilet was full of blood, I felt like I was being continually punched in the stomach, and I was as thin as a twig. I couldn't deal with any of it anymore. I had tried everything I knew, and I was out of options. My doctor's advice was to remove my colon if the condition continued to worsen, because, in addition to the symptoms I was already having, I was also at higher risk for colon cancer. At that point, I thought, if removing my colon was going to relieve my pain, help me gain weight, and save me from cancer, I was going to give it serious consideration.

At that time in my life, everything seemed to be going wrong. In addition to my illness, I had an unsupportive wife, who, among other things, was upset with my emaciated appearance. I had a job I didn't enjoy, and I was over my head in debt. I became so depressed, I gave up hope, and I stopped trying to get better.

I didn't yet know about prayer at that point in my life. I just asked over and over again to no one in particular, "Why me?" I struggled not to become depressed, but as the pain worsened, my mood darkened. I left the bathroom that night and lay down on my bed. I decided that, since the more I ate, the worse I felt, I would stop eating. I wasn't trying to starve myself, but if that happened, I reasoned that it would be better than living with the pain and other issues that came along with my illness.

For three days, I drank only small sips of water but ate no food. On the third day, I realized I was going to the bathroom less often, and there was less blood. I thought this was interesting, but I was more curious to see how much weight I had lost during those three days. I got on the scale. I had actually gained one pound. Wow! Here I was, trying to get better by eating more, when my real healing began by eating less. It didn't take long for me to realize there was something to this eating less, especially during times of pain and inflammation.

The more I thought about it, the more sense it made. When I was a teenager, I sprained my lower back playing in the water at the beach. It was only a minor sprain, but it was still very painful, and I had to stay in bed for a few days, because putting pressure on it would have made it worse. Until the inflammation went down, I had to rest. I began to understand something I had been missing all along: Inflammation is the body's way of saying we are putting too much pressure the body. Just as if I had tried to do jumping jacks on a sprained ankle, eating too much, and not eating the right foods, were putting too much pressure on my digestive tract. Only when I removed what was contributing to the problem did I begin to heal. Years later, when I met Dr. Fred Bisci, he confirmed what I had suspected: "Health begins with what we leave out of our diet."

Poor digestion equals poor health

My experience spurred my interest in diet as the cure for disease. In my readings, I learned that poor digestion is common, and, if not addressed properly, will lead to worse conditions, and that the state of your colon determines the status of your health. To be healthy, you must keep the colon clean and working well.

This information isn't new; it's just often overlooked: Overeating creates poor digestion. Poor digestion creates a toxic bowel. The colon can only handle so much food at any one time. Any amount beyond what it can handle is going to result in serious discomfort or dis-*ease*. Inflammation of the colon, which I suffered from for years, is a result of excess food.

My illness was in a more advanced stage, but everyone should take warning: If you do not address overeating, you also will most likely suffer from inflammation of the colon or worse. I often explain to people today, you may have been able to overeat and have avoided disease up until now, but that's no reason to keep overeating, especially when you have been shown it is clearly not healthful to do so.

If you are overeating, chances are there is inflammation somewhere in your digestive system or other organs of the body. When inflammation occurs, the main function of the body shifts from a digestive mode to a cleansing mode. This cleansing mode is an automatic, built-in garbage disposal that helps keep the body clean. The problem is, after years of using additional energy to keep cleansing, the organs lose their vitality, and there is very little energy left to digest food. The garbage disposal cannot do its job, so it shuts off. The result is constipation, and then more serious diseases, such as IBD or colon cancer, can set in.

Following the advice in this book of not eating late in the day and eating a healthful diet—fresh, organic, raw fruits, vegetables, nuts, and seeds—you should not suffer from inflammation of the colon (or any other part of the body).

Few people today have a clean colon. They suffer from constipation and continue to put more food on top of undigested food. This creates fermentation and putrefaction. Keeping your colon clean, and assisting your body in the digestion of food, is the answer to optimal health. The good news is that we can make that happen. After my own personal experience and my experiences helping hundreds of others, I am convinced we can improve our digestion. By combining foods properly, eating less frequently, and eating fresher foods, we can assist digestion, have cleaner digestive systems, and be healthier as a result. But the best way to health is to temper our eating and eat only during daylight hours.

All about the enzymes

It wasn't too long after I learned the connection between eating less and healing that I was in a health food store and attended a talk on nutrition in the produce department. Up until this point in my life, you would not have found me in any supermarket produce section, because I hated fruits and vegetables. The speaker explained that fruits and vegetables in their raw, uncooked state contain enzymes that assist digestion. I briefly told him about my illness and that the only cure I had found was to abstain from eating. He acknowledged that might work for a while, but eventually I would have to eat or I would waste away. I told him I was scared to eat; any attempt I made to eat caused a setback in my health. On the other hand, I certainly didn't want to waste away.

He said processed foods, cooked foods, and any canned foods or foods that were not fresh would always make my condition worse because the naturally occurring enzymes are destroyed when food is heated or cooked. He assured me that if I ate raw food—fruits, vegetables, nuts, and seeds—I could achieve similar results. In fact, he told me with confidence that if I ate certain raw fruits and vegetables, my condition would heal completely.

This was difficult for me to believe. After all, my doctor had told me raw food would be the worst thing for my condition because my ailing colon would not be able to digest it. Actually, she was partly right: Anyone who was in as bad a shape as I was should not just start eating raw fruits and vegetables unless they know what they're doing; it very well could have worsened the inflammation in my colon. (I would later learn that blending or juicing fruits and vegetables is the best way to consume raw foods until inflammation is reduced.)

The enzyme argument seemed valid to me. According to the speaker at the health food store, a lifetime's consumption of low-fiber foods and foods without live, active enzymes had been a major contributing factor to my illness. Overeating, he said, also contributed to my problem.

Now I was confused. The doctor said one thing; the speaker at the health food store said the opposite. Whom was I to believe? My then-wife helped me make my decision. It was her opinion that the speaker in the health food store had no idea what he was talking about. Since she knew very little about health and had never given me good advice, I knew listening to this man was the way to go. When I informed my doctor of my decision to eat raw foods, she told me I was going to worsen my condition. But the truth was, nothing she had suggested up to that point had helped, so when she gave me her feedback, I felt even more confident that I was making the correct decision.

Until my colon healing, and I could digest raw food in its whole form, the answer for me was to eat raw food in a liquid form, either blended or juiced. It worked like a charm.

Since then, I've spent what seems like every hour of my life studying ways to improve digestion. The more I learn and apply, every time I incorporate a new way to improve my digestion, the better I feel. I am healthier now at age 38 than I was as a teenager. I have more energy, and I'm in better overall physical shape.

As I continue to learn new things about diet and health, I experiment on myself. Once I achieve positive results, I let others know what I'm doing. When they try one of my suggestions and it works for them, it means I'm onto something. Some suggest there is no "one way" for everyone. This is true, because we are all at different stages in our health, and there are many variables that make our own individual bodies unique. However, I think I have found the key to digestive health, and I believe it will work for everyone. It's why I wrote this book.

Less is more.

Eating less for better digestion and health is not a popular idea. We live during a time of excess in all areas of life, especially eating. Most people are not mentally ready to reduce their food intake even when presented with all the facts about the benefits.

Those three days of fasting after I "gave up" on ever finding a cure for my IBD opened my eyes about the role of digestion in health. Like most people, at first I struggled with eating less. Eating the right amount of food didn't happen overnight; it was a process that I had to first understand and then be willing to do. I had to be emotionally ready and mentally sound to stick with it. The more success I achieved, the easier it became.

Raw foods were a big key to my success. But ultimately, if you overeat raw foods and eat them too often, you can continue to harm your body. As the body heals, our chemistry shifts. For this reason, we must continually enhance our diet so we can stay ahead of any possible health issues.

When I began to eat a raw food diet, I could eat what raw foodists call "raw recipes" all day. (A raw recipe is a more healthful version of common cooked recipes. For example, instead of apple pie made with cooked and processed ingredients, a raw recipe for apple pie would call for unprocessed, raw fruits, vegetables, nuts, and seeds for a similarly great-tasting version.) After several years of overeating raw recipes, I didn't feel as good as I had when I first started eating raw. I began to eat fewer recipes. I also combined my foods better and ate less. As I did, I began to feel better. Then, for a few years, I tried eating a lot of mono-meals, such as only fresh fruit, in large amounts. At first I felt great, but, again, I didn't feel well eating so much food. Over time, I realized that less food helped me cleanse better. As my body adapted to less food, my diet had to be continually simplified. Once I reached what I felt was my optimal health, I stayed committed to my new way of eating to keep myself in top form. (It usually takes years of refining the diet to achieve that goal, though, so don't expect to get there overnight.)

I came to realize that eating less food, even in its raw state, was only part of the solution for healthy digestion. For me, the revelation that took my digestion to the next level—and my health along with it—was learning that the times we eat our meals are just as important as the quality and the amount of food we eat, and, most importantly, that it's not healthy to consume food when it's dark outside!

Daylight and digestion

Dr. Fred Bisci once told me that the optic nerve is activated by sunlight, and that stimulation enhances digestion. When the sun goes down, the optic nerve is affected in such a way that digestion then slows down.

I knew this was extraordinary information and became motivated to uncover more about the subject. I spent a great deal of time researching and studying many books on natural health and the best diet for humans. Starting with the Bible, I looked back through history to see what method of eating produced the best results, as well as the most sensible way to eat for ideal digestion.

During my research, I discovered writings by Dr. Dio Lewis, a nationally known health lecturer in the late 1800s. I found his writings on the Internet and liked his information about health and digestion. I wanted to have his complete works on the topic, so I purchased a first edition copy of his book. It was the oldest book I have ever owned, and it contained some of the best information on health and digestion I have ever read. (I've since had this book reprinted and you can get a copy at my website www.rawlife.com) Dr. Lewis's book T*alks about People's Stomachs*, was written more than 130 years ago, yet the information is still astonishingly accurate. As I was reading it, I almost fell out of my chair with joy. The two main points Dr. Lewis makes in his book are about how much to eat and when meals should be eaten.

Here are two quotes from Dr. Lewis that summarize the book very nicely. They confirm everything I believe that promotes ideal digestion:

"'How much shall I eat?' I can't answer that question. You must answer it for yourself. But I had read with earnest interest the advice of the celebrated Dr. Johnson on this point, which is that everyone must observe after dinner, and if he find from his sensations that he has eaten too much, he mustn't do it again. All these opinions and teachings were interesting and helpful, but they didn't help me much just where I most needed help. I knew very well that, as a habit, I ate too much: the only rule which has ever served me is this: On sitting down at the table, take upon the plate all that you are to eat, and when that is finished, quit."

Keep in mind that, back in the 1800s, when the book was written, dinner was commonly served as a noontime meal, what we today would call lunch, or our second meal of the day. (We will discuss this more in Chapter 3.)

"Is it better to eat at noon, and go to work on a full stomach, or to wait till the day's work is done, and then do the eating? My advice to all is this: Eat but two meals a day, and take the last one in the middle of the day. Digestion requires a certain amount of vital force. Early in the day, there is enough to spare after the brain and muscles are provided for. In the middle of the day, while the forces of physical nature are still high and strong, there is enough left to work, and, in addition, digest a good meal. But as night comes on, and the arms of nature are folded, and the man's vital stock is run out, there is nothing left to digest. When the hard day's work is done, it is not the right time to fill the stomach with hearty food. The stomach is as tired as other parts of the body and should be allowed with the residue of the body to rest and not be put at six hours of hard work. With this management, the workingman's muscles and back will remain young much longer, while his brain and vision will be clearer and brighter."

One very interesting note: There was a very popular figure in American history who was encouraged by Dr. Lewis's writings. Lysander Spooner (January 19, 1808–May 14, 1887) was an American individualist anarchist, entrepreneur, political philosopher, abolitionist, supporter of the labor movement, and legal theorist of the 19th century. (He is also known for competing with the U.S. Post Office with his American Letter Mail Company, which was forced out of business by the U.S. government.) As it turns out, Dr. Lewis was a friend of Spooner's, and Spooner is featured in Dr. Lewis' book *Talks about People's Stomachs* (1870).

In the book, Dr. Lewis writes that Spooner, until he was 50, ate three meals a day; then, for nine years, he ate two meals, and, for three years, one meal a day. Spooner suffered a great deal from stomach troubles during his life until the adoption of the one-meal system. With one meal a day, he became as bright and cheerful as a boy, and had skin like a baby's. Dr. Lewis said he did not know another man of Spooner's age so youthful in spirit. (Spooner's success at the one-meal-a-day system convinced him that, if workers of all classes would rise early from eight hours' sleep and digestion, they would be ready for a day's work without eating again until evening.)

Spooner and others subscribed to this one-meal-a-day plan with great success during the 1800s health movement. I agree with the health writers of that time: No more than one or two meals a day are necessary. At the most, eat three meals a day, and the earlier in the day, the better.

Later in this book, I present a three-stage plan to help guide you in your journey to eating the Daylight Diet. Don't worry: I do not expect nor suggest people rapidly go from eating five or ten times a day to only two times. I do recommend, though, that you try to eat only fresh, organic, raw fruits, vegetables, nuts, and seeds, in small amounts, and only during daylight hours. You will find that, as the body becomes cleaner, you'll need less food.

CHAPTER 2

LATE-NIGHT EATING

Just say no to eating after sunset.

As children, we learn and establish our habits based on our observations and then mimicking what we see. Whether they involve eating patterns or a way of speaking, adults' actions imprint messages on young, developing minds. Children are "programmed" in this way, at a young age, to believe that what's popular—what most people do—is the right thing to do and the right way to do those things. We can't know it as children, but, as we become adults, it is much more sensible to use our own personal experiences to guide us to learn right from wrong.

As I observe Americans' eating habits today, it is obvious to me that most people are still thinking as a child: They eat whatever and whenever they want, believing that, if everyone else is doing it, it must be OK for them. Advertisers realize this, too, and use it to create their marketing campaigns.

Everyone wants to be healthy, so why do they mimic the practices of sickly people? Blindly following the blind usually results in some type of crisis. The prudent approach is to pay attention to what works best for your own situation, not someone else's. Nevertheless, that is what child-thinking adults do everyday when they emulate gluttonous eaters: They indulge and enjoy every food to excess, and, once health fails them, they blame others for their dilemma.

Been there, done that.

New York City is often called the city that never sleeps. Another title we can give New York City is it's the city that never stops eating. I've traveled all over the world and have never been to a place that had more 24-hour crowded restaurants in the middle of the night. Not even in Las Vegas would I find the cafes and restaurants so packed at these wee hours of the morning. Being from New York City, I can attest the two most popular places are restaurants and hospitals. It doesn't take a genius to see the connection.

For many years, I was one of the rats in the race: sleeping little and eating all the wrong foods at the wrong times. As a young man, I worked outrageous hours. I desired to be independent early in life, so I took on many jobs. Unlike the average teenager who would get a job after school, I decided to do things differently. My first job started before sunrise, delivering newspapers. Even the birds weren't awake yet. This would not have been so bad if I hadn't just gone to sleep a few hours earlier: After school, I worked at a nightclub and then at a 24-hour bagel store. Sometimes I had more than one job at a time.

After graduating from high school, I worked the "graveyard" shift, 10 p.m. to 5 a.m., at the U.S. Post Office. So, during my teen years, my lunch hour was usually between 2 a.m. and 3 a.m. No wonder that, several years later, I would suffer from a digestive illness. I found out the hard way why they call it the "graveyard" shift.

Soon after I learned about the raw food diet, I became a raw food chef. This was long before my revelation about not eating at nighttime. I first worked at one of the most popular vegetarian restaurants in New York City, Caravan of Dreams, adding raw food recipes to its menu. Later, I helped open the world's largest raw food restaurant in New York City, The Forth Dimension. In both restaurants, the food was so delicious that I found myself eating much more than I should have been. Fortunately, because the food was raw, my digestive condition didn't return, but I came to realize that I had to put my foot down—or, rather, put my fork down—and eat less; otherwise, the digestive issues that had plagued me in the past were going to recur.

I did fine for a while, but a bigger problem was forming: Being in the restaurant business in the city that never sleeps put me on a schedule where I was up until the early hours of the morning. My busy time at work was dinner, serving everyone food, and after my shift, it was my time to enjoy nightlife and indulge. I often ate late at night. There is a saying that you become like the people around you, and I was surrounded by many late-night eaters. Even though I was finally eating less, I ate my main meals later and later into the night. I was just like the people I described at the beginning of this chapter. (That is why I understand them so well.)

At that point in my life, I worked with people interested in raw food, and all of my close friends were raw food eaters. This made eating an all-raw diet easier, of course, but none of us realized how unhealthful it was to eat late at night. We overstuffed ourselves, thinking we were always going to be healthy because our food was raw. We thought we knew all there was to know about diet, and we were going to be an example to the world about how to avoid disease. We couldn't have been more off the mark.

Today, as the raw food movement becomes more popular, I see lots of people making a similar error. I feel blessed to have learned there is more to life than your diet. I've also seen too much to believe raw foods alone can be a panacea. Sadly, many of the people I befriended in those days are no longer interested in a raw food diet. They claim it didn't work for them. Some of them still struggle with the same common sicknesses and lack of energy that they had prior to adopting a raw food diet. The reason the diet didn't work for them wasn't the raw food, but eating too much of it too often, and eating it late at night. Today, they continue to overeat and continue to suffer, and they have yet to discover the correlation.

Going up against the norm

It's not simple to make diet changes in a society that creates many social events around eating, particularly late-night dining.

Even within the so-called health field—the vegetarian and raw food movements—most food-related events are held in the evening. Regardless of the food you eat, if you consistently eat when it is dark outside, your health will never thrive.

Because people are so influenced by their friends and family, they choose to follow the crowd straight to obesity, illness, and disease. The result of late-night indulgence has led to a weight crisis. We now have the most obese people in history, with more people overweight than ever before. Not only is obesity affecting their appearance, disease is also on the rise, because the majority of people are eating way more than they need. In the search for a cure, all but a few wise people run to the doctor for medicine and drugs. This just leads to the same results of more pain and no cure.

Instead of doctors making people aware of their unhealthful addictions, they often give them a reason to make excuses and continue the downfall. Once doctors start to notice a pattern of unhealthful behavior, they invent a disorder and give the public the idea that they don't have control over it. They claim the condition either runs in the family, or it's such a common issue, there is just no cure except to control the symptoms rather than the cause.

I am not blaming doctors for our own faulty behavior; nevertheless, after being in many doctors' offices and hospitals, I have seen how they pay little attention to the connection between food and health, and none between food and eating after sundown.

In my last book, *The Formula for Health*, I wrote about how too much food and lack of sleep are two major causes of disease; I joked that there is something called "sleep-eating." Yes, people eating in their sleep and not even knowing it! It makes a good joke and gets a nice laugh, but the sad thing is that it is true. As scary as that is, one thing I find even worse is that many people overeat late at night and are fully aware of it, but do not attempt to stop.

I once encouraged a group I was speaking to not to eat late at night. I suggested instead of everyone staying up late and eating, why not try getting to sleep early and waking up at sunrise and having a party early in the morning instead of late at night? Nearly everyone thought that was crazy. I find it crazy that people will stay up all night eating and being social, and then they are too tired to get up in the morning.

Since countless people eat late at night and some throughout the night, I sometimes feel hopeless that I will ever convince anyone that late-night eating is harmful to your health. I once read that it's easier to convert someone to a different religion than it is to convince him to change his diet; I have to agree. I once advised a fellow with diabetes that some dietary changes would help him get off insulin. He declared he'd rather take insulin than have to give up junk food. (At least he was honest and not making excuses.)

An addiction or hereditary?

The addiction of late-night eating has grown to be a universal epidemic. Scientists now believe Night Eating Syndrome (NES) affects up to 27 percent of obese people, and roughly 1.5 percent of the general population. (From my observation, it seems more like 95 percent of the population.) It's so enormously widespread that it's now officially a "mood disorder," which, in my opinion, trivializes the problem and relieves the patient of any control over his condition. The patient can now accept the doctor's diagnosis, believing any solution is out of his control and absolving him of any personal responsibility for his problems. This produces fear and stress in the patient, resulting in further late-night bingeing. Then doctors prescribe drugs to treat the issue and not the cause, and, on top of that, the doctor says food must be taken with the drugs, creating even more overeating.

To make matters even worse, doctors are now implying that NES is hereditary. Well, yes and no. If the whole family has the same eating pattern, then they will all suffer from similar diseases. To a doctor, that may be "hereditary;" in my opinion, it's a lifestyle-related condition.

Given that the majority of people will comply with a medical doctor rather than use common sense, convincing someone to modify their diet can be extremely difficult. In spite of this, where there is a will, there is a way, and it's my goal in this book to show you the way. Regardless of your age or ethnic group, your body was designed to digest food best during the daytime. Adhere to the strategy in this book, and before long, you should no longer desire to eat during nighttime hours. Once you comprehend the message and experience the results, living on the Daylight Diet will continue to become more enjoyable, and you'll wonder how you ever wanted to eat late into the night.

CHAPTER 3

DAYLIGHT DIET BY DESIGN

Break with custom, and be healthy.

We have been designed to be on schedule! We have all the tools we need and all the intelligence to know the best schedule for us to enjoy a healthy, long, satisfying life. This book is about that ideal schedule. Of the many ideas and concepts regarding nutrition and what foods are most nutritious for the human body, the majority of people have not taken into consideration the times of eating for best digestion.

As each day passes, we continue to discover new truths regarding health and nutrition, though there is still a great deal to know. Since we don't have all the facts about nutrients and how our body responds to them, doesn't it make sense to focus on the Designer of the nutrients, and the Maker of the body they go into? Only this will assure we are eating the finest foods in the best way possible.

We have been designed to eat certain foods, and at certain times of the day. Just as water in your gas tank will harm the car, bad foods will harm your body. A car is made to run on certain fuel, and so is our body. However, no matter what time of the day you put gas in your gas tank, it won't make a difference. The time you put fuel in your body, however, does make a big difference.

It's also impossible to overfill a gas tank; once it's full, nothing more will fit. Wouldn't it be great if our stomachs acted like that?

The closer we stick to what we were designed to consume, the healthier we will be.

Look to Scripture.

It was our Creator who first separated the salt water from the fresh, made dry land, and planted a garden. He made animals and fish before making even one human being. He provided what we needed before He even created us. If He designed our body and He knows every single hair on our heads, I'm sure he knows what we should eat and when we should eat it.

He created the heavens and the earth, including humans, food, sun, and the moon. The sun and the moon set the schedule we have been designed to follow. The information I share in this book can lead to a healthy life only if we stop watching man's calendar and clock and base our time by the sun and the moon each day. When the sun is up, feel free to eat; when it is down, stop. I can't make this advice any simpler than that! Eat your meals as long as the sun is up, and it is light outside. But when it is dark and the moon is rising, your meals should end for the day. This is the number one rule of the Daylight Diet. If you stick to this important principle, you will see excellent results in your health, energy, sleep—your whole being—because this is how we have been designed to eat. Nighttime is for resting and sleeping.

Custom versus design

Avoiding food at night is an idea that complements everything I've been teaching for the last 15 years about the importance of consuming a high quality diet but eating less often. When you eat high-quality food—raw, organic, fruits, vegetables, nuts, and seeds—you can eat less, because the food you are eating is so nutritionally packed that it satiates your appetite, unlike junk food, which some researchers believe just triggers more eating.

The idea that eating less food makes you healthier is not a new one. Studies of calorie-restricted diets have shown that eating less can result in an overall improvement in your health, strengthen the body to heal disease, and add years to your life. Many health writers of the late 1800s and early 1900s also wrote about the benefits of frugal eating, so it's not a new idea. As a matter of fact, eating late at night has only recently—in the past 150 years—become the norm.

We were designed to thrive under certain circumstances, but we were also created with an amazing ability to adapt to our environment. The importance of this difference is that we can *thrive* for a long time if we live according to the way our body was designed; the farther we transgress from natural design, the more we increase the chances of suffering from disease.

The exciting news is the Daylight Diet—the plan we were created to live by— is so simple, anyone can achieve it. You don't need a lot of money or time; in fact, it will help you save money in the long run. When you are up and awake early in the day, your horizons are automatically expanded. Just think how much you could accomplish if you had more energy and time to get things done. The closer you adhere to the Daylight Diet, the less sleep you will need, because when you eat less, your body is not using so much energy all day on digestion, and you require less rest. So now you can really be free to enjoy life.

You will get so much more pleasure and appreciation for food when eating according to the design for which we were created. More exciting is the enhanced appreciation you will experience for life in all areas, because you will now be living in the way we were meant to live. When you get to that point, it will seem like you have been going against a tide your whole life, but now you can just let go and go with that tide. It's so much easier and fun.

There was a time when even I thought eating the Daylight Diet would be too challenging because I just love to eat. I love to eat more than anyone else I know, so much that when I heard about the popular trend that you should eat many smaller meals throughout the day instead of three large meals, I figured I'd get the best of both worlds: I ate many big meals often.

I've met many obese people in my lifetime, but I never met anyone who ate like I did; when it came to food, I just never felt satisfied. But I had to change my ways, because, even though I loved food at all hours of the day and night, my body didn't. Eating all the time may have satisfied my appetite, but it turned my belly into a pinball machine, wiped out my energy, and made me weak and lazy.

Now, when people tell me they have an eating disorder, or they know they eat too much but can't help themselves, or they don't feel satisfied—whatever the reason—I tell them they're not alone, and that it doesn't have to be that way. They can learn as I did how to enjoy eating great-tasting food that's healthful and satisfying. Now that I eat this way, I never crave food the way I used to.

The divine plan

I often wonder how we ever went from thriving at design to surviving at custom. How did the idea of eating for nourishment become something harmful?

One reason is because today we live in a world where we just never seem to be satisfied with anything; we are always pushing limits. No matter how much we have, we want more, and we want it more often. And the most common thing we want more often is food. The appreciation for the amount and type of food we need has been replaced by wanting food—any kind of food, but mostly the unhealthful kind—to excess.

There was a time when people appreciated any good nourishment they received and never left the table without giving thanks for it. In today's fast-paced world, people don't seem to have time to focus on where the food came from or how privileged they are to be able to get it. (Just visit any Third World country, and you will see an entirely different attitude: true appreciation and thanks given for the food.)

People may say they are appreciative for what they have, but their actions don't always show it. They just eat and run. Fast food restaurants support this fast-eating, unappreciative attitude.

People who take more than they can fit in their bellies and throw away the rest, eating themselves sick in the process, waste a shameful amount of food every day.

When I worked in the restaurant in New York City, I used to take all the leftovers and give them to the homeless people after my shift. Even homeless people wasted food. We just never seemed to be satisfied. We need to learn to truly give thanks for our food and for everything we have.

The healthiest people on record were the ancient Israelites you read about in the Scriptures. During Biblical times, they made sacrifices and prayed twice each day to our Creator, giving thanks for all they had. This happened at the same time every day: the third hour and the ninth hour of each day, usually around 8 a.m. and 2 p.m., depending on the time of sunrise, but never at nighttime. They were not only the healthiest people, but they also lived the longest lives ever recorded. They were vibrant in their later years, climbing mountains, and giving birth. Only when they strayed from the divine guidelines of our Maker did they suffer from the same health problems as the rest of the world.

There are many spiritual communities around the world that shared and continue to share good health also. Just like the ancient Israelites, they eat little, only twice a day, and never at nighttime. The ancient yogis, for instance, and today's Buddhist and Roman Catholic monks all practice temperance when it comes to food. Buddhist monks in the Tibetan tradition eat only once a day, in the morning, and only what they are given by the community.

Who's to blame?

How did the obsession with food and eating many times a day well into the night become the norm? It's all part of the tradition of many communities and countries around the world today to eat in excess. It is really only in the past century that we made indulgence of food a normal practice.

Much of it started as certain social classes who were able to afford food ate more and ate more often than those who weren't as well off.

Social and economic class determined what when, and how much people ate, but today that is no longer the case. Today, different economic, cultural and social classes may have their unique diets, but food within those diets are becoming global, and eating to excess is becoming the norm just about everywhere.

There is now a one-world diet evolving; a fast-food nation. Plus, exotic foods are becoming less exotic and the once strange foods from different corners of the world are now easy to get at our local corner restaurant. With all the differences in diet customs, one thing has sure become the standard around the world: eating many times a day and eating at nighttime.

In reality, people today eat a lot more than just three meals a day; it's more like six or ten times a day if you include snacks, brunches, etc. People always seem to be consuming food. To make people feel good about overeating and eating too often, doctors to advertisers all share a similar message: Eat more. Even many nutritionists today state we need to eat more to get our nutrients. In some cases, that may be so, but in cases of sickness and disease, the answer usually isn't to eat more, but to eat less and at the correct times.

Some people fear eating less, especially people with blood sugar issues or diabetes, claiming they need to eat often to stabilize their blood sugar. A much wiser idea is to eat the right foods at the right times in the correct amounts, and your body will fix everything else. Then there are the claims by the health industry claiming it is more healthful to consume several small meals a day than three larger ones. The problem is, very few people eat small meals, so now we have people eating lots of large meals every day, patting themselves on the back for thinking they are eating healthfully.

Eating many times a day and into the night is so commonplace now that anything less is usually referred to as a "starvation diet." Government child protection agencies would even take a child from their parents if they found out a kid was eating less than their hefty neighbors. I personally know of several families whose children were taken away by child protection agencies because feeding them a raw vegan diet was different from the norm. To add to the insult, the agents who came to take the children were overweight and didn't appear to be healthy.

Let's be animals.

There must have been a time—pre-fire—when it was abnormal to eat after the sun went down. Otherwise, people would have been eating in pitch darkness, and who would do that? Fire brought light into the night, and I'm sure eating at night followed not too far behind.

Now our eating schedule, once controlled by our cultural, economic class, location, and social status, is being replaced by our work schedule, transportation mode, television programming, and marketers. Still, overeating is becoming the norm, and people can't seem to let go of the idea of eating less or giving up their nighttime binges. They are attached to their three big meals and snacking throughout the day. The biggest meal of course is dinner, the evening meal. We have really got it backwards there.

If we observe animals in the wild, we can get a good idea of the ideal ways, times and amounts to eat; not often, not much when we do eat, almost never after the sun goes down (unless they are nocturnal animals, which we are not). We should also take our time and thoroughly chew our foods. I have yet to see a dog bark with food in its mouth, but I see people talking with their mouths full all the time.

Even our pets and other animals in captivity have adopted our unhealthful eating patterns. A wild animal doesn't get right up out of sleep and stuff its face. It hunts and works for its food.

Animals in captivity are awakened by their owners and taught to eat at "feeding time." Humans are awakened by smells and sounds telling us it's our feeding time as well. But it's never healthy to eat right after getting up, and it is not healthy to eat right before going to sleep. If we want to experience better health, we would do much better to return to the way we have been designed to enjoy food.

Naming our meals

As I travel around the world teaching, I have the privilege of staying with many different families. I find it so interesting to see the different ways meals and mealtimes are handled in each family.

If I were an alien from a different planet, and I were plopped into any household in America and heard people taking about their meals, I would think they were talking about people: "Did you spend time eating? Did you spend time with Bobby? Did you remember to meet with Donna? Don't forget you have an appointment with Billy." We have made our meals into something so personal that we actually give them names and make sure we spend time with them every day. We usually don't give our meals a second thought until they are no longer there and withdrawal sets in.

We not only get personal with our meals, but we also have made all our eating customs more personal. People even feel devoted to certain name brands of food and have such an emotional connection to them that they're practically insulted when someone suggests a no-frills, store brand. Just when did meals become so personal that we decided we would name the meals? How have these times and meals changed over the years?

I suggest the ultimate way to eat the Daylight Diet is two meals a day. There was a time when that was the custom. Now we can only look back at it as a passing trend.

When it was "in style" to consume only two meals a day, usually the last meal was taken before it got dark outside. Besides, before electric lighting became popular, only the more well-to-do could have a meal during the nighttime.

The origins of breakfast, lunch, and dinner

It wasn't until the 1600s in Europe that it became customary to consume three meals a day. Breakfast in the morning was the first meal, the second meal was called dinner, usually around mid-afternoon, and a third meal was called supper, usually a light meal in the evening right before sunset. There was no meal called "lunch," just breakfast, dinner, and supper. What happened to lunch? And aren't dinner and supper the same thing?

I too was confused when I first read this, but as I did more research, I found out that during medieval times, dinner was the main meal of the day, served during the middle of the day. Back then there was no such thing called "lunch." I found that interesting, because many of the friends I grew up with in Brooklyn whose parents came from Europe ate according to this pattern every Sunday, enjoying a big meal at lunchtime and having only a light meal in the evening. But other days of the week, they ate like everyone else. (Later, I was thrilled I already understood this, because Dr. Dio Lewis refers to the noontime meal as "dinner" in his writings from 1870.)

In my research, I found the word "dinner" dates back to 13th century England. It was derived from the French word *diner* meaning to dine. Dinner was usually served around noontime or 1 p.m. It was usually the biggest meal of the day. As work demands continued to grow, this midday meal became much smaller and simpler. Only the wealthy had time for a big midday meal. The only time the average person could take the time to sit and eat during the day was when they weren't working, usually on their only day off. You guessed it, Sunday. That explained why many of my friends ate dinner on Sundays around noontime. But what about every other day? And what was the difference between dinner and supper?

When it was customary to eat dinner during the day as the biggest meal, the evening meal of the day was a much smaller meal usually called supper. Supper possibly got its name from "soup," because people usually ate a light meal of soup in that meal because they went to sleep shortly afterwards and didn't want to go to sleep on a full stomach. (Boy, have times changed. It's the other way around now; people seem to enjoy going to sleep on a full stomach.)

By the mid 1800s, as the middle class was able to afford candles and oil lamps, there were more activities taking place in the evening, and eating at night became more common. Also, because people were busier during the day, they didn't have a lot of time to eat a big meal at noontime, so supper gave way to dinner, and people began eating the largest meal of the day in the evening.

Once dinner was pushed back into the evening, people found they didn't want to go without food all day. They wanted a quick meal in the middle of the day. That is when a midday drink became popular. They called it *nuncheon*. Nuncheon was a word for a drink taken in the afternoon between meals, kind of like what we would call a snack today.

It wasn't too long before people began to complain that the drink wasn't satisfying them and they wanted more food during the midday. They began to consume a lump of bread with the drink. Eventually, they combined the *nuncheon* with *lump* and got *luncheon*. That's where we get the name for the common midday meal today called *lunch*—another meal added to the customary two main eating times, plus many other snacks, treats, and desserts added to that.

Meals and times since have varied in different regions of the world, but one thing everyone seems to have in common is nighttime eating, a custom that started only about 150 years ago.

So many meals in a day

So there you have it. That's how we came up with the names

for the common three meals a day and how eating later into the night has become a custom. Eventually, people would get into the habit of eating more than three meals a day. Today we have breakfast, brunch, lunch, snack, dessert, coffee break, dinner, supper, midnight snack...New meals and names just keep coming. It's no wonder people think I'm odd when I tell them to eat only two meals a day.

It has become very popular today for people to eat after dinner. Some people call this a late-night snack or a "midnight snack," even if it's eaten at around 9 p.m. or 10 p.m. Doctors, of course, call it late night eating disorder, or nighttime eating syndrome.

I call it trouble because it results in sickness.

CHAPTER 4

THE HEALTH WRITERS HALL OF FAME

Good ideas gone wrong

Man has transgressed from the Creator's simple eating plan of small amounts of fruits and vegetables during the daytime. Today, man's biggest meal of the day is during the evening hours and consists of heavy meats and other unhealthful foods. Is it possible to return to the simple diet we were designed to eat and regain our health in the process?

Health-conscious people have always tried to persuade others to return to healthful eating and natural methods of healing: Native Americans, and even our Founding Fathers relied on natural methods of healing, using herbs and food to do the job. Even Bible scriptures refer to this. History shows that, during the 1700s, people were preaching about the connection between eating nutritious foods and health. Books were written; people were healed. But something went wrong. Something didn't quite catch on, and now we have a nation of sick, diseased people.

Read, listen, and learn.

We take for granted the value of food. We overeat without giving any thought to what we waste. Food has value. Eaten with wisdom, food will sustain our health and longevity. Only in times of depression do people stop to think about how valuable food really is and how much of a sad thing it is to waste it. Even sadder is that we can—and do—abuse ourselves with food, as if it were a deadly weapon.

Paying no attention to the warnings of obesity and disease, people continue to transgress from health advice. We have become so accustomed to overlooking the value of food, that only a few people make the connection between food, health, digestion, and the Daylight Diet.

We each have a choice to make when it comes to our health. We have all the information and models from the past so we can progress to the future, and it's all based on how we live. It amazes me that we have become so advanced in technology in every area of life, so much that recently a U.S. navy ship shot a small missile and hit its target about the size of a car. This may not seem special until we find out the target was a satellite in space. Meteorologists can predict weather months in advance. All this technology, skill and wisdom, yet man cannot foresee health issues caused by diverging from the designed eating plan meant for health. They could, of course, and are capable of doing so; they just choose not to.

Thanks to a few great men of the past, accurate knowledge about diet and health is still available. We each have the choice to listen, learn, and obey the lessons from these great writers, or to follow the masses and ignore their valuable advice, or worse, to twist their teachings into something far from their original intent, which, unfortunately, has been done time and again, as we'll see.

Hippocrates

The first person who comes to mind is Hippocrates, also known as the Father of Medicine. Growing up, I'd heard about this great man, but never really paid attention until I was sick and looking for a cure. Then I ended up at a place called The Hippocrates Health Institute. I couldn't any longer ignore the important health advice Hippocrates wrote and taught. As twisted as the medical community today has become, the ideas of Hippocrates date all the way back to 400 BC and are still widely used today in the natural health field. Hippocrates's writings are still the foundation of most people interested in natural health. Many physicians today actually take a Hippocratic Oath before practicing any form of medicine, natural or conventional.

Hippocrates has a very special place in my heart, not only because I was healed following the basic health principles he taught, but also because it has become a passion of mine to teach people that food—not drugs—should be our medicine.

At the time when others were blaming their poor health on nondietary factors, Hippocrates came along to show disease was the direct result of poor diet, bad habits, and environmental factors.

Hippocrates based his teachings and therapeutic approach on the healing power of nature. He was one of the first to teach that the body contains the power to heal itself, and that the physician should simply help it along. He didn't like the idea of prescribing harsh drugs because he believed physicians could harm a patient if they mistakenly gave him the wrong substance. Considering one of the leading causes of death today in hospitals is mistakes by doctors, we can see how far we have transgressed in the field of health.

What did Hippocrates have to say about The Daylight Diet, or at least the idea of the timing of eating certain foods? He often mentioned seasonal eating: Winter foods are heavier and sustain us longer when the days are shorter. In the warmer months, the food is naturally more cooling to the body and much lighter on the system. Summer produce has much more liquid than dense, winter produce. Hippocrates addressed these issues often, and I have found out that they perfectly go right along with what I have learned and teach about The Daylight Diet.

Of all Hippocrates's teachings, the one that appeals to me most is his focus on the dangers of overeating: "If they who have been accustomed to one meal a day should chance to eat two, they soon grow dull, heavy and thirsty." He wrote about the health problems you could suffer when you take in more food than the constitution will bear. He also wrote about the importance of exercise and the correct combinations of food, today known as food combining. (If you read Hippocrates, you will also appreciate his poetic style. Here's an example: "A variety of foods, discordant in their nature, should not be indulged at one meal, because they make a disturbance and create wind in the bowels." I am a writer, but it takes a gifted poet to come up with such a beautiful way to say that if you don't eat right, you get gas.)

Hippocrates made more important contributions to the advancement of medical science than anyone in history. His instructions seem to us now simple enough, but for the period in which he lived, they were little short of miracles.

After Hippocrates, the next significant physician was Galen, a Roman of Greek origin who lived from 129 to 200 AD. Galen was of the Hippocratic School and revived the practice of Hippocratic medicine.

Galen

Galen was a prominent and legendary (even in his time) philosopher, and medical researcher who produced more writings than anyone of that age. It's estimated he wrote almost 600 works on anatomy, physiology, and logic, although fewer than 200 of them survive. He could discuss Plato, Aristotle and the Stoics, but above all, he paid homage to Hippocrates.

Galen, like many of us, was not very healthy at a young age, but his discipline for preserving health helped him survive and thrive 140 years. Today, we strive to reach an old age and feel blessed if we can make it to 90; so, when you find a man who lived to be 140, you know he knew his health stuff and was putting it into practice. His teachings about preventing disease can be summed up with this quote: "A man, whose body is clear from every noxious humor (waste) that can hurt it, is in no danger of contracting any illness, except from external violence or infection."

His other advice included suggestions we still hear from doctors, nutritionists, and modern health experts: Exercise, and eat plain and simple food that is easy to digest. And, by all means, do not eat more than you need.

There's that idea again: temperance in all things, especially diet. Seems so simple, but we have drifted so far from what is good for us. My next example is someone I've been researching about 15 years now. He is the perfect example of the amazing healing power of the human body when we let it do its job and we don't get in the way by overindulgence.

Luigi Cornaro

His name is Luigi Cornaro, and he was born in 1464. Cornaro's writings are so inspiring to me and helped me understand the value of temperance in eating. His story begins as a young nobleman who ate rich food until he was 35, at which time he grew ill. His doctor fortunately knew what he was talking about and advised him to stop eating so much and to eat just small amounts of easily digestible foods and wine. As Cornaro's health improved, he soon realized that stuffing himself had caused long-term health problems. He believed it was time for him to take control of his health.

Cornaro began to live what he called the "temperate, moderate, or simple life." In addition to having written political satires and plays, he also wrote, in 1558, Trattato de la vita sobria, or Treatise on the Simple Life ("simple" meaning, in this case, moderate, or frugal). He reduced his food intake, cutting it down to 12 ounces of solid food a day, divided into two meals, with 14 ounces of light wine, also divided into two servings. Within a few months on his new and essential diet, his health improved remarkably. Shortly after his new life of wisdom, clarity, and health, he married, became father to a daughter, and eventually had 11 healthy grandchildren, the joy of his advanced years.

Cornaro believed we should eat the best quality and most easily digestible foods, but in small amounts. (Sounds like The Daylight Diet!) He enjoyed excellent health on this regimen for more than 65 years. Most days, he ate one egg yolk, vegetable soup, coarse, unrefined bread, salads, and small quantities of locally grown fresh seasonal fruits and vegetables. He sometimes ate a little meat (all cattle were free range and grass fed in those days), eaten in very small portions and only on special occasions; neither fish nor chicken agreed with Luigi, so he avoided them. He also drank slightly fermented wine. It's important to know that, in those days, wine was not bottled as it is today, but was kept in barrels; and since it was consumed in the same year the grapes were harvested, it contained only a fraction of the alcohol of today's wines.

At age 85, even though he was very happy and satisfied with the way he was eating, his "well-meaning" relatives began to implore him to eat more. Finally, to stop their incessant badgering and to appease them, he increased the amount of his food from 12 to 14 ounces. He also started drinking a little more wine, going to 16 ounces a day from 14 ounces. Within 12 days, he developed a high fever. He knew exactly what had brought it on—an increase in food and drink—and he returned to the smaller amounts he had been used to when he was healthy. His health returned. At 95, Cornaro had all his faculties intact; his judgment, memory, and joyful spirit were undiminished, and he continued to live healthfully on the smaller quantities of food and drink.

Cornaro was very active until his death at 102. His health never diminished over the years. He had all his senses, no memory loss; even his eyesight and hearing had grown keener with the years. In his nineties, he studied singing and horseback riding and to the end of his days, led an active life. To the last moment, he believed that small meals were the perfect guarantee of physical, mental, and emotional happiness.

It's important to note that all food was of higher quality in mid-16th century Europe than it is today. It was entirely organic, and there were no packaged foods, no processed foods, and no supplements. None of the plants native to the Americas (coffee, cacao, tobacco, cane sugar, corn, peanuts, potatoes, tomatoes, etc.) had yet been imported, and it wasn't until the 19th century that wealthy Europeans had become largely addicted to the first four. Imagine a world without sugar, coffee, chocolate, tobacco, potatoes, tomatoes, or corn! There were no distilled beverages, no sodas, no processed candies, no white flour, no white rice. Medications were all natural, herbal remedies; there were no petroleum products, no plastics, no factory farming, etc. The world was still truly green, not commercially and environmentally challenged.

On the subject of intemperance in eating and drinking Luigi wrote:

"We should live up to the simplicity dictated by nature, which teaches us to be content with little, and accustom ourselves to eat no more than is absolutely necessary to support life, remembering that all excess causes disease and leads to death. I conclude that excesses in eating and drinking are often fatal.

"The safest way to attain a long and healthy life is to embrace sobriety, and to diet oneself strictly as to quantity.

"The two most important rules of eating and drinking, which I have ever been very scrupulous to observe, is not to take of either, more than my stomach could easily digest, and to use only those things which agree with me.

"Neither is it necessary that all should eat as little as I do or not to eat of many things from which I, because of the natural weakness of my stomach, abstain. Those with whom all kinds of food agree, may eat of such, only they are forbidden to eat a greater quantity, even of that which agrees with them best, than their stomachs can with ease digest. The same is to be understood of drink. The only rule for such to observe in eating and drinking, is the quantity rather than the quality; but for those who, like myself, are weak of constitution, these must not only be careful as to quantity, but also to quality, partaking only of such things as are simple, and east to digest.

"Strict sobriety, in eating and drinking, renders the senses and understanding clear, the memory tenacious, the body lively and strong, the movements regular and easy; and the soul, feeling so little of her earthly burden, experiences much of her natural liberty. The man thus enjoys a pleasing and agreeable harmony, there being nothing in his system to disturb; for his blood is pure, and runs freely though his veins, and the heat of his body is mild and temperate."

Cornaro was a true trailblazer, and his story proves the capabilities of the human body. His message is simple and would help anyone today who is looking to improve his or her health. Another special thing about Cornaro was that he was not a doctor. He was just an ordinary person with a lot of common sense.

John Wesley

The more I studied health, the more I was led to the Bible, where it speaks of fresh fruits and vegetables, practicing temperance in all things, especially diet, and where gluttony is considered a major sin. As I look around churches today, I see church leaders overweight, unhealthy, and providing foods to the people that were never mentioned in the Garden of Eden. I discovered this was just another area were people started out with good, simple, sensible ideas about health and confused the message we get today.

From the beginning of Biblical time, we were supposed to eat healthfully and at the right times. It is what we were created to do. In my research, I found a man who taught this very message more than 200 years ago.

John Wesley, an Anglican cleric and Christian theologian who was the founder of the Evangelical Methodist movement, was preaching a message about the connection between our health, our lifestyle, and diet based on Scripture to support his views.

He authored a number of books on health reform. His recommendation for the best of health was moderation in food and drink.

Sylvester Graham

Less than 100 years after Wesley, people continued to overindulge and consume unhealthful foods. The majority of people were sick and getting sicker giving very little attention to diet as a means of healing. In a time when many people were eating meat and other heavy, low-fiber foods for breakfast, Sylvester Graham came along to advocate whole grains, vegetarianism, and temperance in all areas of life, especially in eating. If his name sounds familiar, it's because you see it often today if you visit the supermarket cookie aisle. Graham was the inventor of the Graham cracker. Today, though, it is little more than a junk-food cookie amongst the dozens of other junky snacks that line the grocery shelves. At one time, though, it was a wholesome food. A little history lesson can show you how a great idea turned into an unhealthful product.

Sylvester Graham believed that dense bread made of coarsely ground, whole-wheat flour was more nutritious and healthful than what was being offered at the time. He also believed chemical additives used in many breads of that time were harmful. He set about inventing something more nutritious and came up with a cracker-like break. During that time, it was a much more healthful version than what it is today, and it is yet another example of how we have moved backward instead of forward.

Today, graham crackers are the very thing Graham was trying to convince people *not* to eat: refined flour, sugar, and other stimulants. When I go to the store and see chocolate-covered graham crackers, I shudder at how this wise man's message of health has been lost in time.

Graham inspired many people to join in the health movement, but we have continued to go in the wrong direction. We have to get back to the garden, get back to his message about the purity of food. His points were simple, and they worked. Unfortunately, graham crackers are just one example of someone taking a brilliant health message and turning it into an unhealthful version of the original, for profit.

To a degree, the message of the health movement today can be summed up in the story about the Graham diet. We have a wonderful health message that works, that makes good health sense, but people got away from it, and they are suffering as a result.

Dr. Dio Lewis

Soon after Graham, someone came along who made quite an impact in the world of natural health. His name was Dr. Dio Lewis, and he became a leader in the Christian temperance movement. In fact, it's his message and the way he presented it, that really resonates with me. My conclusions on health, diet, and temperance so closely matched what he wrote. I don't agree with his choices and ideas about what constitutes good quality food, but the timing and amounts he suggests are right in line with The Daylight Diet.

His real name was Diocletian Lewis but was usually called Dio. Lewis was a temperance leader who practiced a form of natural medicine known as homeopathy. Lewis learned about health from a modern medical standpoint but chose to use natural methods.

In the 1850s, Lewis became a nationally known lecturer on health reform. He taught many of the same things as Graham, but he also prescribed eating only two meals a day and suggested that it would be more healthful not to eat at nighttime. Lewis was the first health reformer I came across in my research who advocated those two important prescriptions for health. Though the majority of the ideas for The Daylight Diet came before "knowing" Lewis, once I read his books, I knew his writings would be a big help in getting out my message. I was so excited by what I read that I purchased a first edition book of his from 1870 called *Talks about People's Stomachs*. (I believe the book is too important to just tell everyone about. I want everyone to read it so they can get a good foundation for the Daylight Diet. For this reason, I had his book reprinted. You can order it at my website www.rawlife.com.)

Like many of the other health writers of the past, Lewis's message never really caught on with the mainstream. While he was advocating control over eating habits, people just wanted to eat more and more. Plus, he understood the importance of sunlight to digestion and that it just isn't healthful for people to eat when it's dark outside. You will see that I quote Lewis many times in this book, because I believe his message was right on the mark, and more people need to get it.

James Caleb Jackson

Graham had quite an impact on James Caleb Jackson, an abolitionist and lecturer during the mid 1800s. Like Graham, Jackson developed a food that would help transform people's diets. Unfortunately, also like Graham's, it would be transformed into something far from what he had in mind.

Jackson originally wasn't interested in health until stress got the best of him and he decided to seek natural methods of healing. During those days, hydrotherapy, or water treatments, was very popular, and Jackson believed that hydrotherapy had cured him of his ills. He was so enthused that he became a doctor so that he could treat others with hydrotherapy. He eventually bought a spa in Dansville, N.Y., on the site of a mineral spring. It became world famous, and people began flocking to Jackson's spa in search of health and healing.

Eventually, Jackson began to understand the role of diet in health and illness. He began removing certain foods from the spa menu—meat, coffee, tea, alcohol, and tobacco—and promoting a diet of fresh fruits, vegetables, and unprocessed grains.

His real claim to fame came in 1863, when he invented the first whole-grain breakfast cereal and named it *granula*. (Yes, granula. We'll get to the other one in a minute.) Jackson's granula was pretty bland tasting, but people ate it because it was high in fiber, and fiber was all the buzz in those days. Unfortunately, since people usually care more about the taste of something than the health of it, it was just a matter of time before the popularity of granula would blow over.

But granula wasn't Jackson's biggest impact on the health movement. He reached more people through the fame of his students than through his own teachings. Two of his most popular students became very popular health teachers: Seventh Day Adventist leader Ellen G. White and John Harvey Kellogg. (Kellogg would later modify the granula recipe and market it as his own, changing the name to *granola* to avoid litigation.)

Just as Graham's healthful cracker had been turned into something it was never meant to be, Jackson's bran-based granula/granola is no longer the healthful breakfast food it once was. Although still promoted as good for you, most granola today lacks the bran it started with, is high in oil and sugar, and may be drenched in honey and contain M&Ms.

Ellen White

Next we get to the real prize of Mr. Jackson's work, Ellen G. White. In my opinion, Jackson's well-presented health teachings have reached thousands through White's books. White started a movement that led to the founding of the Seventh Day Adventist Church. In visions from God, White was told the importance of following the right principles in diet and care of the body, and of the benefits of nature: clean air, sunshine, exercise, and pure water.

For 50 years, White spoke and wrote about the importance of a healthful, balanced diet. She reached hundreds of thousands of people in her writings, which to this day are considered some of the best health books ever written, and her teachings were almost identical to my Daylight Diet. I have read many of her writings, and I continue to reread them for support and inspiration. Here are some excerpts from her works:

"A failure to care for the living machinery is an insult to the Creator. There are divinely appointed rules which, if observed, will keep human beings from disease and premature death."

"Respect paid to the proper treatment of the stomach will be rewarded in clearness of thought and strength of mind. Your digestive organs will not be prematurely worn out to testify against you."

"It is possible to eat immoderately, even of wholesome food. It does not follow that, because one has discarded the use of hurtful articles of diet, he can eat just as much as he pleases. Overeating, no matter what the quality of the food, clogs the living machine, and thus hinders it in its work."

"In most cases, two meals a day are preferable to three. Supper, when taken at an early hour, interferes with the digestion of the previous meal. When taken later, it is not itself digested before bedtime. Thus the stomach fails of securing proper rest. The sleep is disturbed; the brain and nerves are wearied; the appetite for breakfast is impaired; the whole system is unrefreshed and is unready for the day's duties."

"After the regular meal is eaten, the stomach should be allowed to rest for five hours. Not a particle of food should be introduced into the stomach 'til the next meal. In this interval, the stomach will perform its work and will then be in a condition to receive more food."

"Regularity in eating is of vital importance. There should be a specified time for each meal. At this time, let everyone eat what the system requires and then take nothing more until the next meal."

"Regularity in eating should be carefully observed. Nothing should be eaten between meals: no confectionery, nuts, fruits, or food of any kind. Irregularities in eating destroy the healthful tone of the digestive organs to the detriment of health and cheerfulness."

"It is quite a common custom with people of the world to eat three times a day, besides eating at irregular intervals between meals; and the last meal is generally the most hearty and is often taken just before retiring. This is reversing the natural order; a hearty meal should never be taken so late in the day. Should these persons change their practice, and eat but two meals a day, and nothing between meals, not even an apple, a nut, or any kind of fruit, the result would be seen a good appetite and greatly improved health."

"Three meals a day and nothing between meals—not even an apple—should be the utmost limit of indulgence. Those who go further violate nature's laws and will suffer the penalty."

Sounds like the Daylight Diet, doesn't it?

John Harvey Kellogg

White may have never created a breakfast cereal, but as destiny would have it, one of the members of her new church was John Harvey Kellogg, who, with his brother, Will, of the now famous Kellogg family, founded the world's leading producer of box cereals and convenience foods.

The cereal business has come a long way since the days when Kellogg, a medical doctor, opened a health retreat/spa for people to relax, heal, eat well, and learn. Besides diet, he offered other holistic methods, with a particular focus on nutrition and the benefits of enemas and exercise.

There are a lot of interesting stories about the serendipitous invention of corn flakes, and of the partnership and eventual split of Kellogg's relationship with his brother, Will, in 1906, over what direction to take with this new, well-received health food. (Will took off on his own and founded the company we know today.) In addition, they created another biscuit similar to Jackson's, but by all accounts it tasted much better. Then they further insulted Jackson by calling it by the same name: Granula, which they changed to granola when Jackson threatened to sue. That was the beginning of the end of this one-time healthful food.

Other companies got on the granola bandwagon, and what was once a high-fiber breakfast cereal became what we know today. Like most "health foods" produced by multinational corporate entities, something is lost in value once it becomes world-known and mass distributed.

C.W. Post

One of the visitors to the Kellogg spa was a man named Charles William Post, also known as C. W. Post. In the late 1890s, he would create one of the world most popular cereal lines, including Post Grape-Nuts.

But these products became more about profit than health and led to the line of unhealthful cereals both companies—and many others like them—are producing today.

Arnold Ehret

During this time in Germany, there was a health teacher who was gaining a lot of fame by healing people with diet. He was Arnold Ehret.

When Ehret was 31, he was diagnosed with Bright's disease, an inflammation of the kidneys. Doctors all over Europe examined him; each one diagnosed his disease as incurable. Ehret turned to alternative medicine for help. He visited health sanitariums throughout Europe and Africa in a quest to learn about holistic healing. He discovered that simply eating less not only made him feel better, but he found that he also gained strength and vitality. Eventually, he credited his fruit diet and fasting for healing both his heart condition and his kidney disease.

Ehret opened a sanitarium in Switzerland and became widely known for curing thousands of people whose diseases had been labeled "incurable" by physicians. He was known for his long periods of fasting, anywhere from three to seven weeks, and for his fruitarian diet. In 1909, Ehret wrote a book called The

Cause and Cure of All Human Illness. He became one of the most popular health lecturers in Europe, and, in 1914, brought his knowledge to the United States, where he also lectured and wrote his seminal treatise on diet and health called The Mucusless Diet Healing System. ("Mucus" was his term for phlegm.) He died at age 56 after a fatal head injury resulting from a fall.

Ehret's book is still an inspiration to people who are passionate about health. His diet is expertly planned to transition the patient from a toxic diet to a combination of fasting and a healthful, high-quality diet. His "Formula for Life" sums up the state of health in a brilliantly simple equation that easily shows us how good health is created. I will discuss Ehret's formula in a future chapter. His "Formula for Life" and the tenets of the Daylight Diet are, I believe, the keys to understanding and achieving great health.

Ehret believed that eating too many mucus-forming (toxic-forming) foods was the cause of most disease. He talks about vegetarians overeating starches and other unhealthful mucus foods being even more harmful then poisons such as meat, alcohol, coffee, and tobacco, even in small amounts: "This is the solution! Even these habitual toxins are less harmful than stuffing oneself regularly with good old 'comfort' foods."

Ehret often quoted Sylvester Graham's saying, "A drunkard can get old, a glutton never" when speaking about the issue of overeating being even more harmful then drinking.

Ehret's book was one of the first health books I read about eating less food, and only twice a day, for better health. To this day, I refer to it often and suggest everyone read it.

It appears he did suggest skipping breakfast, but I believe that was misinterpreted: I think he was suggesting not eating right after arising and giving the body a chance to wake up. My Daylight Diet suggests waiting several hours after waking before eating the first meal. Ehret also never wrote about not eating at nighttime but suggested eating two times a day and not going to sleep on a full stomach.

Again, we have a great health teacher who wrote simple books about eating less and achieving great health that people for the most part do not do because they have been brainwashed into believing they need to eat a lot to be healthy. Arnold Ehret did a great job proving them wrong.

My good friend Alvin Last, founder of the Ehret's Club, has translated Ehret's writings and has kept them available. Ehret's first book, The Cause and Cure of Disease, written in German, was discovered after Ehret's death. Alvin had the book translated into English, and it is one of the best health books I have ever read. You can join the Club, buy Ehret's books, and find out other great health information at www.arnoldehret.org You can also purchase Ehret's books on my site www.rawlife.com.

Dr. William Esser

I had read so much about people using the fundamentals of what I came to call The Daylight Diet, but it would be a while before I began meeting people who actually followed those fundamentals. The first was Dr. Will Esser. I had the privilege of meeting Dr. Esser at his fasting health ranch in Lake Worth, Fla., where he had supervised an estimated 30,000 fasts. Dr. Esser lived a healthy life, playing tennis up until his death at 92 years. He preached temperance in eating and observation of nature's laws. He wrote many articles on the topics and wrote a book, Dictionary of Natural Foods.

I saw firsthand how Dr. Esser's energy surpassed most people half his age. His diet was basic and very simple: two fruit meals and one vegetable meal per day. Most of the food was fresh, grown on his property. He himself rarely went on a fast because, he told me, he didn't have to because he didn't overeat.

According to Dr. Esser, eating a good variety of fresh fruits and vegetables was important, and he often suggested limiting ourselves to a few certain types of food is not in the best interest of good nutrition.

In an interview I did with Dr. Esser, he said overeating and over-indulgence are the two biggest health errors people make that can shorten and alter the quality of life. Plus, he said, we should not go to bed until our digestive systems have completed most of their work for the day; otherwise, digestion will interfere with our sleep, both the quantity and the quality.

He didn't eat much food, because, he said, the body cannot deal with large amounts of food. Our body struggles to get rid of excesses any way it can; if we overindulge, it simply can't keep up, and toxemia builds up.

The following are some of Dr. Esser's teachings. They are taken from an article he wrote in 1958 that was reprinted in the January/February 1998 issue of Health Science magazine. The magazine is published by the National Health Association (www.healthscience.org), and this is used with permission:

The power of fear

'The result of such teaching is the building of fear complexes, which reduce vitality and lower health standards, and is a prominent reason why other nations point to America as a country of sick people. Sadly, there is shocking truth to this belief. The average American has developed 'the habit of being sick.' Seeking cures from curers is the tragic national pastime. Cures are as elusive and unreal as mirages. But the palliation and subsequent impairment of vital organs— and the surgical mutilation—are very real and lasting.

"The time is long overdue for thorough renovation. The causes of fear must go. Man has nothing to fear except himself and his disease-building, life-shortening habits. Years ago, when the microscope enlarged tiny organisms to a size that made them look ferocious and dangerous, a wave of fear swept the land. It was decided that these caused most of our diseases and, as a consequence, a sterile existence was frantically sought after by all who wished to be healthy. Today, the fear of germs is mostly a thing of the past. But another phobia, more mysterious but less tangible—the 'virus,' has taken over to explain disease.

"Illness results from man's own violations and indiscretions, his own sins against himself. When he ceases to make himself sick, he becomes immune, and disease no longer exists. John H. Tilden, M.D., once wrote, ' All the cures which have been invented by man are boomerangs that have returned to do him evil.'

Freedom of will

"Man has freedom of will. It is about time that he becomes aware that his destiny is of his own choosing. The knowledge of health and its maintenance is not exclusive with a small chosen group of people. Nor is the knowledge too technical for the average mind to grasp. Man's willingness to allow someone else to think for him has almost caused him to lose his self-protection.

"The animal kingdom has its claws, teeth, beaks, and other instinctive defenses for protection and for securing food for young and self. But man has his mind, which gives him dominion over everything else on Earth. He has opened many doors and unlocked many mysteries with his mind. Unfortunately, he knows more about things outside himself than he knows about himself. The results of this ignorance, plus lack of self-control, are sickness, pain, and premature death. And the accumulated sequences of crime, perversity, war, and a decaying society are the by-products of this ignorance. Unless man learns to know himself, he will destroy himself.

Knowledge is strength

"Sickness is unnecessary. Those who possess good health should know why they are well. If the only reason they can give is that they have always enjoyed good health and that their ancestors were good specimens of longevity, they have no reliable knowledge with which to keep the good health they possess. Their good health potential and sound constitutions can easily be frittered away.

"The fact that parents and grandparents lived to a ripe old age gives one a fine feeling of security but is very much like an athlete resting on his laurels. Unless he continues to train and maintain his achievement, he will soon find his records toppling. The asset of long-lived forebears can be offset easily by the rush and worry of modern business, or by a frantic social pace, which outdistances that of our fathers by at least five to one.

Challenges we face

"Today, there are many advantages over previous decades, but there also are many disadvantages. The machine age, with its push button existence, enables men and women to achieve many things with great efficiency. But it does nothing to relieve the grueling pace and tension that goes hand and hand with it. The nervous and digestive systems, brain, and heart are taxed far beyond their endurance. In order to keep up with the demands of competition, tobacco, coffee, and other drugs are relied upon to stimulate flagging nerves and functions. The man is wise who from time to time withdraws from the insanity of today's graceless living for somber contemplation of true and eternal values.

Requirements of life

"Natural laws are unchanging. They govern each of us. To push beyond individual requirements in working, eating, sex, and pleasures—without sufficient allowance for restorative rest to replace what has been spent—promotes much suffering and earlier death.

"It is not the aim of Natural Hygiene to invalidate the definite advances which man has made since the beginning of time. It is, however, necessary to point out the flaws in civilized living, and the false security which comes from depending upon the physician for health, rather than upon obedience to natural law.

Common sense

"Common-sense care of the body is all that is necessary; not some peculiar kind of food or vitamin preparation, nor a disagreeable asceticism. Fanaticism is unnecessary. Live in keeping with natural law, determine to be moderate, and poise of mind and body will be the natural result. The difficulty lies in disentangling oneself from the web of conventional and synthetic living. Cold, analytical investigation is the key."

This information is just the tip of the iceberg. William Esser gave a lecture every Sunday at his health ranch for free. I was blessed to hear many. His teachings of simplicity and moderation have remained with me. He was such a nice man and so wise. I also remember him and his great teachings. He really did walk his talk.

Dr. Stanley Bass

Another person I met who shared so much information with me over the years is Dr. Stanley Bass. Dr. Bass has been a natural hygiene doctor since the 1950s in the New York area, supervising more than 30,000 health recoveries using diet and fasting. (See his website: www.drbass.com.)

My research on temperance in eating led me to Dr. Bass, who has done much study and research on the topic. His age speaks for itself. Dr. Bass is almost 90 and attributes his long life to temperance while eating. For many years, he ate one meal a day. Today, he eats mostly blended foods so his body won't have to use a lot of energy on digestion. I learn from him every time we find time to have a conversation.

I've since met a good number of people on the Daylight Diet; one teacher of it even wrote the foreword to this book, my friend Tonya Zavasta. But of all the people I've met, no one has been able to explain the whole health picture and importance of daylight and darkness better than Dr. Fred Bisci.

Dr. Fred Bisci

Dr. Bisci has a Ph.D. in nutritional science and has run an active, pioneering practice in New York City for more than 40 years. Dr. Bisci has a knowledge and appreciation for the body's biochemical processes and how food and other variables relate to them.

Dr. Bisci's clinical experience and knowledge has repeatedly demonstrated to me that a commitment to lifestyle change is the key to optimal health. He has concluded that there is a correlation between a long-term diet of unprocessed foods and the slowing down of aging. "If we feed the body the correct combinations of fresh vegetables and fruits along with some cooked meals, the body can heal itself. When we exclude toxic foods from our diet, we release our body's God-given ability to always return to health." I've spoken to Dr. Bisci many times about the book you have your hands, and he confirms my belief that the most important thing people can do right away for overall healthy is to stop eating at nighttime.

I've been blessed to have traveled the world with Dr. Bisci, and, other than his own family, I have probably heard him lecture more than any other person. I am so pleased that he finally published his book, *Your Healthy Journey*, which sums up his teachings and beliefs. I suggest everyone read it and study it. If you really want to continue your knowledge about health and diet and improve your digestion to achieve great health, I highly suggest visiting Dr. Bisci's website at www.Fredbisci4health.com.

The health advocates of the past and present are doing their best to present a message that will keep us healthy. Even with all their great efforts, one look at the world we live in shows that their efforts are going against a tide of people not wanting to take responsibility for their own health. It's so simple: Eat fresh foods, eat less often, eat smaller amounts, and eat only during the day. It doesn't get much easier than that.

Others have put these principles to practice with great success, teaching the same core message of temperance while eating. Seek, and search, and you will find. The information is out there. It's up to you to take action, and make it happen.

CHAPTER 5

BREAKING THE NIGHTLY FAST

What you need to know about breakfast.

Before I learned about the health benefits of not eating later in the day, I often ate until late at night. I usually finished my last meal around 7 p.m., but then I'd have a snack around 9 p.m.

This means I would go until about 8 a.m. the next morning without food. That's about 11 hours, during which the body is digesting, healing, and getting the deep sleep the body needs. As we have discussed throughout this book, the later we eat at night, the less healing and the less cleansing will take place.

The digestive system takes at least two or three hours to completely digest a light meal of healthful food that's been eaten the correct way, meaning: fresh, raw, ripe, fruit or vegetables chewed well and eaten under no stress. It will take the body much longer to digest the food if any of those elements are missing. Even a small, junky snack, such as a piece of cake or a couple of cookies, can take up to four to five hours to digest. Bigger meals will obviously take even longer, and, if there is meat or other animal products in the meal, it could take even longer than that.

If you eat a junk food snack at 9 p.m., your body does not complete digestion of that snack until many hours later. That gives the body far less time to rest. Also in this common case, if you have to get up at 7 a.m., you're giving the body still fewer hours to do its cleansing, which can take place only after digestion is completed. Even if you ate a healthful snack at 9 p.m. that would digest more quickly than a junk food snack, you are still interfering with resting, healing and cleansing time. The bigger or more unhealthful the meal, the more time it takes.

Now if your last meal was a nutritious meal finished around 3 p.m., and you intend to get up the next morning around 7 a.m., you'll be giving your body up to 14 hours to rest and heal. That's many more hours than if you ate your last meal or snack at 9 p.m.

It should start to make sense now why we sleep so much better if we don't eat late at night and feel so much better in the morning after a good night of sleep. I felt tired for years when I woke up in the morning. No wonder! Now the earlier I consume my last meal of the day, the better I feel, and it dawned on me that I felt so good because I was actually fasting for so many hours each night.

I have to laugh when some people tell me that going without food for more than a few hours is not healthy. Don't they realize they do it every night? We all fast every night, the longer the better

The nightly fast is also where we get the name for our first meal of the day: breakfast, meaning literally "break fast." Like any fast, our nightly fasts should be ended, or "broken," at the right time and with the right type and amount of food; otherwise, the benefits of the fast are lost. But this is what happens when people jump out of bed and eat a big, junky breakfast. Anyone who understands fasting can tell you this is a harmful practice. The Daylight Diet helps make it simple and easy for you to understand and to pick the right foods in the right amounts at the right time.

Breakfast then and now

History shows that breakfast was usually the smallest meal of the day—unless you were wealthy. Usually it consisted of some fruit, toast, or some sort of porridge. If you could afford more, your servants would prepare a big meal, and you might dine for quite a while, maybe the whole morning. In the mid 1800s, the breakfast meal went from luxury to necessity as health writers started touting the benefits of eating fiber in the morning. People were now not just eating breakfast because they were treating themselves to a big meal; now they began to do it for health reasons, believing it was important not to miss.

Today, one of the most common mistakes people make is starting off their day by rushing through their breakfast meal, grabbing a quick muffin or bagel on the way to work or school or errands. It's always a good idea to take your time while consuming food.

Another mistake is eating as soon as you wake up. Sometimes I think a better name for breakfast should be "fast break." Today people run to the nearest McDonald's or other fast food store if they don't have time to grab a cup of coffee and a donut for breakfast at home. Before fast food, microwave ovens, and other quick cooking methods, people had to take time to prepare their breakfast. That gave the body a chance to fully wake up before it had to deal with food again.

People should relax and enjoy their breakfast, but they usually don't have time because they went to bed late the night before, overslept that morning, and woke up too late to have a peaceful and relaxing meal. For that reason, many people just skip breakfast completely, making up for it by eating more throughout the day and night.

No matter what time you eat your first meal, the first food (or drink) is technically a breaking of a fast. If you don't have time to enjoy a meal at home, it's fine to skip it until a few hours later; however, rushing through it later is not the answer either. You want to eat when you have time to sit and relax and enjoy it.

My discoveries have led me to believe the ideal time to eat the first meal is the beginning of the third hour of daylight each day. This is assuming you are waking up at the ideal time: daybreak each day or perhaps an hour before sunrise. Then give the body a chance to wake up fully by exercising or getting some sort of work done before eating. Working up an appetite means just that: working! Then sit down to a healthful meal that is not rushed or eaten under stress. That is the ideal situation.

For years, I didn't eat breakfast because I just wasn't hungry in the morning. I realize that was because I ate my last meal so late at night. I tell people it is best to get up early and they say they are not morning people. That's because you stay up late at night. Get to sleep early, get a good night's sleep, and you will become a morning person. If you do not like to eat in the morning because you're usually not hungry, don't eat late at night, and you will have an appetite in the morning.

People who just grab something quick (and usually sweet, dessert-like foods) for breakfast, will be snacking by lunchtime. Snacking adds extra food on top of the undigested food that was eaten only a short time before and weakens digestion, creates fermentation and putrefaction, and stresses the body overall. I find it interesting that "desserts" spelled backwards is "stressed." If you partake in desserts at any time—especially right after a meal, it will greatly stress your digestive system.

Of all the health tips I can give you, there are so many advantages to starting your day when the day starts—at sunrise. By getting up at sunrise, you'll have more time to get done what you need to get done before the end of the day. One of the major reasons people do not succeed at the Daylight Diet is because they wake up too late in the day. I have found the most relaxing thing is to be up and out when the sun comes up. It is so beautiful, and you can enjoy breaking your nightly fast in the most healthful way.

CHAPTER 6

QUALITY AND QUANTITY

Late-night eating has got to go.

People tell me often that eating brings them so much pleasure and that they do not want to limit what makes them feel good. Well, I did not write this book to take away your pleasure, but one of the purposes of this book is to take the focus off how *you* feel for a moment and think about how your *stomach* feels *all* the time.

How would you feel if every time you were about to fall asleep at night someone woke you up? Or what if you were up many hours and so tired all you wanted to do was get some rest, but the people around you made sure to keep you busy? These are just some of the things we put our stomach through when we overeat and eat late at night.

Yes, eating is pleasure, but think about this: The more you please your stomach, the better you will feel. Most of our physical internal illnesses are connected to the condition of our colon. Disease starts in the colon. Whether it's a cold, flu, headache, rash, inflammation, tumor or anything else that causes discomfort in the body, they are all a result of a dirty, overworked colon as the result of an unhealthy digestive tract as a result of overeating and eating at the wrong times.

One of the keys to health is having clean, healthy blood. When digestion is not allowed to work as it should, the colon does not eliminate as quickly as it should. This creates a buildup of waste. If not properly and quickly addressed, this waste ends up in the bloodstream in the form of toxic gas. Just as the water in your house may run dirty because the reservoir has not been cleaned, the colon is the reservoir of the body. Your blood is the "water of life."You must keep clean and healthy.

The type of food you eat is a big reason your colon may not be clean, but a bigger reason is the amount of food you eat and how many times a day you eat it. It is far worse to overeat, even high quality food, than to consume low quality foods in small amounts. In other words, it's the quantity that does far more damage than the quality.

Don't get me wrong:The quality of the food matters, because if the food you eat does not nourish your body, you will crave more, and then you will most likely overeat.

Because people eat low quality food, people often actually gradually starve themselves, even if they eat a lot. Starvation isn't just a lack of food; it is also a lack of nutrients or the inability to access those nutrients. A high quality diet—fresh, raw fruits and vegetables, nuts and seeds—means we can eat less. Problems arise when we try to satisfy our hunger based on eating the amounts we became accustomed to on a low quality diet. This is often the reason that people remain sick or sometimes even get worse when they switch to a high quality diet; they are simply eating too much, and the stresses on digestion are the same as if they'd been eating low quality food.

Although we can't be in control of what happens to the food once we swallow it, there are things we can do prior to swallowing that can make it easier for our body to digest our food:

- Make the right food choices: Raw, fresh fruits and vegetables, nuts, and seeds should form the basis of our diets.
- Prepare food properly. Avoid foods that are fried or made in a microwave.
- Chew thoroughly to make it as easy as possible for the body to digest the food we've eaten. Each bite should be liquefied and mixed well with your saliva before swallowing it.
- Eat during the daytime only and never when it's dark outside.

- Never eat while stressed. No matter how good the food or what time it is consumed, if you are stressed while eating, it's not going to digest well.
- Eat two meals a day.

Two a day

Our ultimate goal should be two meals a day and only during the daytime. There is no reason why everyone can't live perfectly healthfully on a two-meals-a-day diet. (Three would be the limit. It's not as healthful as two, but still much better than the eight to ten times a day most people eat.)

Again, try to look at it a different way: Studies show that the less you eat, the longer you live. The longer you live, the longer you will be eating, so the more you will be able to eat. Now that's looking at the bigger picture. As you space your meals out more wisely, over the years your organs will be less stressed and become more efficient.

You won't starve on two meals a day as long as they are nutritious. In this country, "hunger" is often a hunger for the habit of eating—rather than hunger for food—and that is not true starvation.

Heavy lifting.

But don't people who do manual labor or work hard need more food than two meals a day? Let me tell you a story.

When I wrote my first book,The Raw Life, I lived on the fourth floor of a building in Brooklyn, N.Y. There was no elevator, but I was very fit, and I exercised all the time, so going up and down stairs wasn't a problem for me. When my books arrived from the printer, the truck driver said the contract stated he didn't have to carry them up to my apartment; he only had to leave them outside the building.

I had no one to help me, so I had to bring them up myself—all 160 boxes, 32 books to a box, and each box weighed about

35 pounds. On an empty stomach, I carried all the books up the stairs to my apartment on the fourth floor. On some trips, I took two boxes at a time. It took me hours, but I'm being honest when I say I didn't break a sweat. (OK, I was a little sore the next day, but that's all.)

When my next book was printed, I made sure it was in the contract that the driver (and a helper, if needed) deliver the books to my apartment, not just to my building. I also ordered half the amount so I wouldn't run into the same problem. When the truck pulled up, two big guys got out. They looked strong, so I was confident they'd get all my books upstairs.

They each took one box up the stairs while I waited at the truck. They weren't looking so good when they came back down. After about four trips, they were covered with sweat and said they needed a break. They were breathing pretty heavily and could not finish the job, so I had to do it.

I called a friend, Dr. Fred Bisci, whom I told you about in Chapter 4. He was in his 70s at the time, but I'd never met anyone with more endurance. He came over, and together, he and I schlepped the boxes of heavy books up the stairs. Neither one of us broke a sweat. You see where I'm going with this: If a man in his 70s who eats only a raw, vegetarian diet and eats only two meals a day has more stamina than two big truck drivers, I don't think you have to worry about not having the energy to do your job.

Be a trailblazer.

As Dr. Bisci explains, it's a real challenge for someone who is eating the standard American diet to suddenly reduce his food intake: The person is not used to it, and neither is his body, and sometimes this does more harm than good if done too quickly. But if time is on his side, he can make a gradual adjustment to a lighter diet, and his body will adjust accordingly. Whatever the case, we have to learn to eat high quality food and less often to be healthy, and, as long as our mindset is in the right place, and we understand health, the Daylight Diet works for everyone.

I give examples of foods to avoid later in this book, but of all the harmful foods we consume and the alarming number of times we consume it, nothing will harm your health more quickly than eating during the evening and the night. The earlier your last meal in the day, the better. So yes, if a person didn't want to cut out all the junk food, as long as they didn't eat it during the later part of the day, they'd be better off. Everything begins to slow down as the body gets ready for rest and sleep.

When I was writing this book, I would ask people to try the Daylight Diet; just about everyone said, "No way." They just couldn't. However, I did find a few people who already had been doing it for years, and who have had tremendous success. I've always said, "If one person has done it, that proves it's possible. If no one has done it, be a trailblazer."

Recent health literature admits we need to eat less. Few of the writers, if any, talk about the optimal times to eat.

My friend and raw food health author Tonya Zavasta, in her book Quantum Eating, also talks about her experience of not eating after 2 p.m. for years and how it has kept her looking beautiful, healthy, vibrant, and young. She defines "quantum eating," as an advanced level of a raw food lifestyle, and the most healthful way to eat. Quantum eating is eating a 100 percent raw food diet, twice a day, and only in the first part of the day. If you think it's almost impossible to lay off food at nighttime, this way of eating must seem not very practical or desirable to you. But it is practical. Think of all the reasons for eating healthfully: Losing weight, gaining energy, being able to focus mentally.

Not eating late at night is certainly the best way to lose weight and keep it off, but as Zavasta puts it in her book, "The very fact of eating less frees the mind from the unnecessary obsession of deciding what and when to eat next. The average person spends a great deal of time in thinking about, shopping for, preparing, and eating food. Worse, they do it three to five times a day! Add working, watching TV, and sleeping, and your life is pretty well shot without ever having had an idea, let alone an original one."

People are sicker today than ever before, and people are eating more food more often than ever before. You might think you'll just eat less, since that's a big part of the Daylight Diet. Well, that will help for sure, but not eating at night will help you more. Fasting is the greatest method of healing our body, and when you take a sick person's food away and give them rest, they heal. Remember, we already do it: We fast every night when we go to sleep until we wake up in the morning.

All I'm suggesting is that you stop eating earlier than you have been. This way you can consistently let the body do its healing/protecting job it was designed for without getting in the way.

PART II

Digestion and the Daylight Diet

CHAPTER 7

LET THE SUN SHINE

It's sunlight that really gets digestion moving.

Obtaining and maintaining good health is actually pretty simple: Abide by the laws of nature that manage your body; straying from these principles will result in damage to your body.

Think of it this way: Take the law of gravity. There is no altering that law, and denying it can have disastrous and even tragic results. As a result, no one questions the law of gravity. We don't have to justify it, because we can witness how it works.

The correlation between the sun and digestion is another example of one of the laws of nature. Exposure to sunlight promotes easier digestion. Digestion and assimilation become weak and imperfect if we are not exposed to the direct rays of the sun on a daily basis. Defying this natural law will not result in the same immediate damage as breaking the law of gravity, but over time, serious damage will take place.

How does it work?

There is a direct connection between the optic nerve and digestion. When sunlight hits the optic nerve, electrical impulses are transmitted, activating many processes of the body, including digestion. Nerve impulses send messages that tell the body to produce certain enzymes, gastric juices, and other processes of digestion. Similar to the act of chewing, when the optic nerve is stimulated by sunlight, the digestive organs prepare for food.

When the sun goes down, there is less light stimulating the optic nerve, and digestion slows down. This declaration does not sit well with people who take pleasure in eating late at night. As I acknowledged in the introduction, people will continue to look for excuses to indulge in their addictions, but ignorance of divine and natural law is why numerous people encounter disease. This is not a mystical, New Age idea. Just as God breathed air into man and gave him life, He designed our organs with capabilities no man-made machine can fully reproduce.

Please do not misunderstand: I am not claiming that digestion grinds to a halt once the sun goes down. What I am saying is that eating after the digestive system slows down in the evening goes against the laws of nature and will result in a decline in health.

Dr. Dio Lewis, in his book T*alks about People's Stomachs*, tells a story about one of his patients, a Mr. P., who complained about stomach problems. According to Dr. Lewis, dyspepsia (the medical term for stomach upsets) was written all over his face, shown in his movements, and heard in his voice. The patient, a local merchant, told Dr. Lewis he could no longer work because of his troubled digestive system. The first question Dr. Lewis asked was about his diet. Mr. P. explained that he was very educated about the subject and his diet was all right. The next question Dr. Lewis asked was if he exercised. Mr. P. revealed he spent several hours a day exercising. Dr. Lewis followed with a question about his sleep, and Mr. P. said he was in bed every night at 9 p.m. and was awake every morning by 6.

Dr. Lewis was a brilliant man, asking Mr. P. essential questions about diet, exercise and sleep, three issues that always need to be addressed when a person is dealing with illness. Mr. P. could not understand why he was having digestive issues since he seemed to be doing everything right; his wife was worried he may even have cancer, because nothing seemed to help him, and the problems kept getting worse.

Finally, Dr. Lewis asked him if he worked in a sunny office. His workplace was pleasant, Mr. P., said, but it did lack sunlight. Dr. Lewis replied:

"Mr. P., that is the cause of your cancer! Your work place needs more sunlight. No plant or animal can digest in the dark. Try it. Plant a potato in your cellar. Now watch it carefully. If there is a little light, that potato will sprout and try to grow. But surround it with the best manure, water it, do the best for it, only you shall keep it in the dark, it cannot digest and grow. See how slender and pale it is. Now open a window in another part of the cellar and notice how the poor hungry thing will stretch that way. Or give the stalk a little twist and see how it will lie down. It has no strength to raise itself again. No matter how much of the best food and drink you give it, it can't digest. The process of digestion, the great function of assimilation can't go on without the sunshine."

Dr. Lewis told Mr. P. that he already had excellent habits, but that, if his workplace had a flood of sunlight, he would be better within one week and completely well in a month. He suggested Mr. P. move his desk in front of a sunny window, even if it's sunny for only three or four hours a day. He assured Mr. P. that, within three days, his digestion would improve. He gave Mr. P. this excellent example:

"Mr. P., did you ever go into the country late in the summer? Of course you have been. Well, did you ever notice, where grain is growing in an orchard, that the part under the trees is smaller than that outside and away from the trees? The land is actually richer there. For years, the leaves have fallen and decayed under the trees, but, notwithstanding this, the wheat is only half size and never fills well. Now what is the difficulty? The sun shines upon it more or less. Yes, that is true, but that under the trees does not receive as much sunshine as that away from them. That which is thus partly in the shade can't digest so well.

"Have you never noticed that the only grapes that become perfectly ripe and sweet, that the only peaches that take on those beautiful red cheeks, and offer that luscious sweetness, are those that are on the outside, entirely uncovered by the leaves and perfectly exposed to the sun? God's laws are the same in the animal world. We all need to baptize ourselves freely in God's glorious sunshine. People who don't get good sunshine are usually very pale."

These examples by Dr. Lewis are excellent ways to show how we need the natural light of the sun to help us digest our food.

Cleansing versus digesting

Once the sun goes down, and the moon appears in the sky, the body switches from ideal digestive time (day) to ideal cleansing time (night). Just as the sun's rays support digestion, the moon (and its gravitational pull) supports cleansing. Just as the moon has gravitational effects on oceans and rivers, it also influences the body to release water and toxins. The fuller the moon, the more cleansing takes place. Cleansing is slowed down if the toxins that are supposed to be released during the night are held back by a heavy meal eaten within a couple of hours of bedtime. The key is to sleep on an empty stomach. This advice can sometimes worry people, because no one likes to experience hunger. So I have to assure them that, when the body is working the way it should, and we are eating at the correct times, our appetite will naturally diminish as the moon rises and the sun sets. You won't "go to bed hungry."

One reason many people seem to be hungry at nighttime is due to the stimulating effects of artificial lighting, entertainment (TV, videos, loud music, and the like) and eating at the wrong times. All of these things will cause us to lose the natural intelligence of the body. Artificial lighting plays havoc with our body cycles, negating our natural eating schedule. Television and video games stimulate our brains so that we can't rest. Together, they actually make us hungry at times we should be abstaining from food. (They also have a stimulating effect on the body that can wipe out our energy and add to stress. The darker it gets outside, lights should start to be dimmed and, even better, turned off.)

Still don't believe the effect of light on the body? Consider sunglasses. I once read that wearing sunglasses outside actually enhances a person's chance of getting sunburned. Sunglasses block the sun's rays from reaching the optic nerve, tricking it into thinking that it is dark outside. This causes the body to produce less of a protective skin coating, increasing the risk for sunburn and even skin cancer. After reading about this, I decided to try it: I have now stopped wearing sunglasses, and now I never get sunburned, and I don't need sunscreen (though I'm very careful not to overdo sun exposure). The human body is designed so incredibly that it works with all the elements of nature, especially the daylight and darkness.

The unknown unknowns

One of my favorite parts of Dr. Lewis's book is a lecture he gave, denouncing patent medicines. A famous doctor, a manufacturer of a famous blood purifier, was in the audience and interrupted his speech with several complicated questions in a loud and passionate manner:

"Famous Doctor: 'Do you know what you are talking about?'

"Dr. Lewis: 'Well, I confess there are some things about it, which I never could understand.'

"Famous Doctor: 'Well, sir, I have given 40 years to the study, *the profoundest study* of the human system, and I should like to put a few questions to you, sir, if you have no objection, sir.'

"Dr. Lewis: 'Speak on.'

"Famous Doctor: 'Will you tell me what a *fever* is?'

"Dr. Lewis: 'I don't know.'

"Famous Doctor: 'Will you tell me what an inflammation is?'

"Dr. Lewis: 'I cannot.'

"Famous Doctor: 'One more question. Will you be kind enough to inform us, whether you can explain the philosophy of any kind of disease, whatever—the simplest thing you can think of—say, a slight headache?'

"Dr. Lewis: 'I have to confess that I cannot.'

"Famous Doctor: 'Well, that's all I want to know; and now I will take my family and go home; and I advise my friends and neighbors to go home, too, and read the story of the babes in the woods; they will find that a good deal more scientific and instructive than this lecture.'

"The world-renowned manufacturer of a medicine, which by cleansing the blood of all impurities, eradicates every vestige of disease from the entire organism,' grandly rose and left the room, and a considerable number left with him.

"To the remaining crowd, Dr. Lewis said: 'Friends, the doctor did not half sound the depths of my ignorance. I not only do not understand the nature or philosophy of any disease whatsoever, but I really know nothing of the nature of the vital principle, in its simple or natural manifestations, saying nothing of it when it is complicated by disease. But worse than this, I know nothing of the philosophy of health or disease in a blade of grass, even, or in one little cell in that little blade of grass.

"In truth, I must confess, for myself, that I have always been sitting before the curtain. Never have I been permitted a single peep behind it into that secret green-room where nature manipulates the ropes, wires, and springs which she employs in producing the great drama *of life*.

"I think this strange, arrogant determination to know all, in physiology, has proved a fatal obstacle to progress in these studies.

"He, who will humbly sit at the feet of nature, may learn all that is important he should know. The Good Father has hidden nothing beyond our finding, which is essential to our welfare and happiness.

"But *life*, which is probably identical with God Himself, is not for our mortal ken.

"We return to the subject under discussion. While no mortal will ever comprehend the *vital* force, while the *philosophy* of digestion must, in its *essence*, remain among the hidden things, all that need be known about the conditions on which this great, pivotal function of our earthly life may be maintained at its highest is quite within reach of the earnest inquirer."

Dr. Lewis's answers may mislead you into thinking that he doesn't know much about medicine, but he had a medical degree from Harvard University. He also authored some of the most intelligent health books I've read. His perspective on healing is brilliant:

"Let us stop putting on airs and frankly acknowledge that not only are we utterly ignorant of the *life* principle, but that the essence of *every force* is absolutely hidden from us.

"Let us modestly study such facts and make such deductions as come within the range of our capacity and leave it to such distinguished and magnificent greatness as to the Above to dive into the profoundest depths of the mysteries of the Creator, to fully comprehend it all."

Since Dr. Lewis wrote his book in 1870, many health mysteries have been solved, though many still remain uncovered. One of Dr. Fred Bisci's favorite sayings is, "We don't know what we don't know."

There are four requirements for survival: air, water, sunlight, and nourishment. Eliminating any of these for a certain period will affect the body negatively. Water, fruits, vegetables, chewing, and sunlight help us receive these requirements. Nature provides the ideal foods found in the soil, vines, and trees. We have teeth to chew our food, and we have the sun to supply us with heat, vitamins, and light. It is no accident that they all fit together like a puzzle.

Staying close to nature ensures our good health. You may be able to replace real teeth with false teeth and stay healthy, but you cannot substitute processed "food" for real food or artificial lighting for sunlight and expect to stay well. The replacement of fresh produce with processed foods has increased the rate of disease during our lifetime more than any time in history. Trying to mimic nature is not beneficial to the body and will create a decline in health. Every part of creation has a purpose and adheres to a schedule. Trying to change this or substitute for it will not produce the same results as nature herself.

CHAPTER 8

NO MORE BEDTIME SNACKS

The importance of rest and sleep to digestion

Good digestion is the key to good health, and the digestive system works best during daylight hours. I keep repeating this, because most people don't understand how important this is to their health since our culture continues to encourage us to eat our largest meal of the day at night, followed by a snack just before bed.

True, digestion is most efficient after a meal—if you're relaxed and not very active—but going to sleep for the night after a meal is never a good idea. It leaves the digestive tract with a good amount of work to be done throughout the night while you're trying to sleep, meaning you're not getting the kind of restful sleep you need.

Rest up

Always rest after a meal, and do not disturb the mind with thinking.
—Aurelius Cclsus, 1st century Roman physician.

When I worked in an office building on Wall Street in New York City, there were often days the weather was not cooperative, so I stayed inside and ate my lunch at my desk. At the time, I didn't mind much, because I got paid for having lunch at my desk. However, when the weather was good, I couldn't wait to get outside. After eating, I would sit or lie in the park and feel the sun on my skin and rest for a little while before going back to the office. I always felt better afterward. In the wintertime, though, I'd rush right back to my desk, and somehow, I never felt as good.

Even if you don't have a lot of time, a brief rest after a meal is better than none at all. Another wonderful way to assist the body in digesting a meal is to also rest before the meal. Too often, people go from a busy workload right to eating and then immediately back to work. I have found taking a short walk before running to and from the lunchroom will aid digestion.

Dr. Lewis mentions in his book about a Dr. Harwood, who noted the effects of a rest after eating. He fed two dogs. After eating, one dog slept while the other ran and played. Two hours later, both dogs were killed. The dog that had slept had completely digested his food; digestion had barely begun in the stomach of the dog that had been running and playing.

Eating while nervous or stressed is never wise; digestion will be most efficient when you are calm, so it is always a good idea to relax before and after eating. The Bible tells about all of Israel eating during certain hours each day and praying before each meal. I personally try my best to read a scripture in the Bible or some other type of uplifting, encouraging message, and pray about it for a while before sitting down to eat. It shifts my mind off work and prepares my mind and body for food. I always feel better when I do this. Occasionally, if I eat while rushed, I do not feel I digest the meal as well. I have learned if you don't have time to relax before and after a meal, it's a good idea to just skip the meal completely. Even a 15-minute break can be great for your digestion. Dr. Lewis notes in his book:

> "In my own personal experience, I have always observed that an hour or an hour and a half of rest before dinner contributes more to the completeness of digestion than the same rest immediately after eating."

Digestion will be more efficient when a person is less active before or after the meal; hence, the caution not to swim or run after eating. In some cultures, a nap in the afternoon after eating is common, although you should do this only to help your digestion; falling asleep because you ate too much food isn't exactly what I'm referring to, because it is never wise to indulge in so much food that you are dozing off at the table.

Eating our last meal earlier in the day leaves us some time to rest after we eat and digest most of our food before we go to sleep for the night. Instead of eating in the evening, try taking a nice walk. That way, when everyone else is just sitting down to eat, you will be finished with your meal and getting ready for good quality sleep because your stomach won't be full. Dr. Lewis said:

> "The time given to the meal itself should be ample. Every minute saved to business by hurrying the eating is an investment, which instead of paying a profit, involves a great loss."

"OK," you're thinking, "I'm with you so far. But where am I supposed to find the time for all this resting?" Obviously, the more often you eat, the less time you will have to rest. Plus, if you eat late at night, there isn't sufficient time to rest before you have to go to bed. There is only one true way this can be done: Get up early, go to bed early, and eat fewer meals.

Sleep deeply.

There is a difference between sleep and deep sleep, or sleep and good quality sleep. Just because you are lying in bed with your eyes closed doesn't mean you are sleeping as well as you can be or should be. We have all experienced where we didn't get to sleep easily, and we tossed and turned all night. In the morning we just didn't feel rested. Then there are other times we sleep so well we awake well rested and felt great. Much of that had to do with the quality of sleep you got.

Deep cleansing and healing mostly take place during the later stage of sleep. For this reason, it is essential to get this deep, restful sleep every night. The more you eat before going to sleep, the longer it will take the body to get to this important stage because your body can only get there once the last meal is completely digested.

Most people are inclined to focus on the amount of sleep they get and not the quality of the sleep, which is more significant. Of the stages of sleep, the last stage is when deep healing and cleansing take place. These days, many people commonly reach this stage only briefly during the night. They may spend a good deal of time in bed, but they are not well rested when they get up in the morning, and it's because they eat too late at night.

Following the divinely designed eating and sleeping plans will establish the greatest opportunity to get the optimal amount of the deepest stages of sleep.

Regardless of what you may have been told, the times we eat have a huge impact on our health, because all health comes down to the amount and quality of sleep we get. Eating a good diet and at the right times is the best way to assure ourselves the needed time to rest each night. In addition to not giving your body enough time to get deep sleep for healing, eating before going to sleep can also contribute to weight problems, which are a common cause of insomnia.

In his book, *Talks about People's Stomachs*, from 1870, Dr. Dio Lewis gave this great example of why it is important not to eat too close to bedtime.

"A man goes hunting. He takes with him a hearty lunch but comes home at dark, tired and faint. He is exhausted all over and very naturally feels faint and gone at the pit of the stomach. His remedy for this is to fill the stomach with steak, fried potatoes, hot biscuit and, butter. The next morning he can hardly stir and makes certain deductions with regard to hunting which would not have been seconded by Nimrod. It was not the hunting which did the mischief. The system had been inflamed in every part by the attempt to digest an enormous supper (late night meal) with an exhausted stomach. The result was, the whole body was inflamed and so was sore all over. He thinks it was the long walking; but if he had gone to bed after drinking a cup of tea and or milk, he would have risen in the morning so bright and happy that he would have formed quite a different opinion of the healthfulness of hunting.

"When the hard day's work is done, it is not the right time to fill the stomach with hearty food. The stomach is as tired as other parts of the body, and should be allowed, with the residue of the body to rest, and not be put at six hours of hard work (digestion).

"Workingmen should eat their last meal at twelve to one o'clock, and take nothing after that but a cup of tea and milk. At first, and perhaps constantly, a pint of this gently stimulating and nourishing drink may be taken at the close of the day. With this management, the workingman's muscles and back will remain young much longer, while his brain and vision will be clearer and brighter.

"I must not forget to remark further upon a point which I think will occur to many of my readers.

"It is this. Is it better to eat at noon and go to work on a full stomach, or to wait till the day's work is done, and then do the eating? Several physiologists have advised, on physiological principles, to wait till the day's work is done, rest for an hour, and then take the principal meal of the day. This seems specious, and not a few have adopted it. But it is a mistake. As this is practically a very important point, I will give it a careful consideration.

"One may eat a very hearty breakfast, and at once engage in hard work: no harm comes of it. No one even advises against going to work after breakfast. It is the dinner which is discussed in this regard.

"Why is this so? Obviously, because digestion requires a certain amount of vital force. Early in the day, there is enough to spare, after the brain and muscles are provided for. In the middle of the

> day, while the forces of physical nature are still high and strong, there is enough left to work, and, in addition, digest a good meal. But as night comes on, and the arms of nature are folded, and the man's vital stock is run out, there is nothing left to digest with.
>
> "He began the day with ten gallons of vital force. At noon there were five gallons left. At night the force is all drawn off. He hasn't a pint left. With some little refreshing, gentle stimulus, like a cup of weak tea, he must go to bed, and after eight hours' sleep, will have his ten gallon vessel full and ready again. Now he starts with his ten gallons of nerve force for another day. It takes three gallons to do his work during the forenoon, and two gallons to digest his breakfast. During the afternoon he consumes three gallons for work and two to digest his dinner. Night finds his vessel empty, but ready to fill again during the eight hours of sleep.
>
> "My advice to all is this: eat but two meals a day, and take the last one in the middle of the day."

Dr. Lewis has given us excellent advice. Now, I don't suggest taking a cup of milk before going to sleep, but we have to remember this was written in 1870, and milk was not considered as harmful as it is today. In those days, milk was most likely raw, fresh from the local farm, and drug free. Today, I would never suggest anyone consume store-bought milk. As for tea, if you feel hungry after work or in the evening hours, taking an herbal tea that does not contain caffeine is an excellent idea.

In my own health research, I have found Dr. Lewis's conclusions to be true. Your stomach should be as empty as possible before going to bed for the night. I know countless people who eat late at night within a few hours of going to sleep. They claim they cannot fall asleep on an empty stomach, but they also profess that, no matter how many hours they sleep, they always are tired in the morning. Eating at the right times of day would more than likely solve that problem for them.

I usually finish my last meal several hours before sundown. Depending on the season, this is usually between 3 p.m. and 5 p.m. Sometimes, after my last meal later in the day, I might enjoy a cup of herbal tea. In the summertime, I sometimes have lemonade, made of lemons, water, and stevia as the sweetener. But I do not eat after sunset, because eating later in the day always affects my sleep in a negative way. I have unpleasant dreams, toss and turn all night, and feel very tired in the morning. When I limit my meals to two a day, at earlier times, my dreams are pleasant, and I sleep much better. I wake up feeling refreshed and vibrant.

Another thing I have come to realize is when I eat late, I always require more sleep than when I eat my last meal earlier in the day. When I eat my last meal earlier, I also always feel much more mentally focused and physically active the next day; my whole mood is much more joyous.

I don't even like to drink water before going to bed because getting up to go to the bathroom can interrupt my deep, Stage Four sleep. I have found if you drink enough water throughout the day, there is no need to drink water before going to sleep. If you desire some water upon retiring for the night, make sure it is a very small quantity. The exact amount a person can drink without having to get up to go the bathroom in the middle of the night varies from person to person, but usually, any more than eight ounces will affect your sleep. Pay attention for a few nights so you'll soon be able to tell how much water you can drink before bedtime without having to disturb your sleep. The best time to drink most of your water is upon rising in the morning and between meals throughout the day. Never drink with your meals; water dilutes the saliva and prevents digestive enzymes from working as well.

Raw food author and natural beauty expert, Tonya Zavasta, has come to the same conclusion. In her book, *Quantum Eating,* about health and natural beauty, one of her health tips is not eating or drinking many hours before going to bed for the night. Tonya does not eat or drink water after 2 p.m. She appears to have discovered the fountain of youth. Tonya looks many years younger than she actually is and is vibrant and glowing. One of her key messages: Do not let food and drink interfere with sleep.

Of all the tips I've learned from Dr. Lewis, this passage from a chapter in his book sums up the requirements for good health and long life:

> "Every person of remarkable longevity, whose habits I have studied, retired to rest at an early hour. He may have transgressed other laws of health; for example, he may have used spirits and tobacco moderately; but I have read of no long liver who habitually sat up till a late hour, and I may add that, among them all, I have never read of a large eater.
>
> "Eat right and sleep right, and you have the two fundamental conditions of health and long life. Establish these two sources of life as fixed habits, and, if you get drunk once a month and smoke five cigars a day, you may, notwithstanding, live a long life in the enjoyment of good health. But sit up in furnace-heated rooms till eleven o'clock, and eat the quantity and quality of food consumed by people who believe in a short life and a merry one, and you may rest assured that the yearly trip to the mountains, a month's guzzle of Saratoga waters, and the attentions of a fashionable doctor, all put together, will fail to save you from early wrinkles, early loss of sight, premature gray hair, and a short life.
>
> "Then, do you ask me how you can reach eighty-five in the enjoyment of all your faculties?
>
> "I reply, go to bed at nine o'clock and eat twice a day a moderate quantity of plain food."

Early to bed, early to rise

To successfully achieve the Daylight Diet, you have to go to bed early and get up early. It's the only way you can eat your meals at the best times, rest before and after the meals, and go to bed without a full stomach. This will ensure that your body reaches cleansing during the deep stages of sleep, and that digestion doesn't keep you up or wake you up at night.

If you arise too long after sunrise, your body misses valuable digestion time. As we talked about earlier, sunlight stimulates the optic nerve, which sends out signals that cue the digestive system. The longer you sleep, the less time your optic nerve can be stimulated by sunlight, and the less time you have during daylight to digest your meals. Plus, most likely you will eat after sunset because, when you wake up later, you usually eat your last meal later. Sleeping late puts you into a rut very quickly. You also usually have a hard time getting to sleep at a sensible time the next night when you've slept later in the morning.

To determine the perfect time for sleep, keep in mind nature's method of telling time rather than man's clock on the wall. We may need that clock on the wall to schedule business meetings and live in the world; however, remember it is an instrument of this world and not the natural one. If you want supreme health and energy, get in the habit of living your life around nature's clock: the sun and the moon.

The optimal time to go to bed is sundown or soon after. Yes, I know, this is next to impossible nowadays; a realistic goal would be 9 p.m. or 10 p.m. These days, most people are just getting their biggest meal of the day on the table at sunset if not later. Then they make plans to go out for the evening. But remember that, once the sun goes down and the moon appears, our body rhythms slow down, and eating after sunset is out of sync with nature.

Good health requires we get a certain amount of sleep each night. Arising early in the morning while still getting the necessary amount of sleep can only happen when we get to bed several hours before midnight. This helps you obtain important rest while preparing you to be refreshed and ready for your daily activity when you rise. People today are often too tired to get out of bed in the morning, due to late-night eating and staying up late. Because of work and other responsibilities, most people are usually forced to awaken well before their body has completed its job of cleansing. Lack of sleep is one of the prime causes of sickness, because the digestive system hasn't yet finished its job for the night.

Beware the night.

People overeat and overindulge in all things more often at night than during the day. Just pass most restaurants at nighttime:They are much more crowded than in the daylight hours. After the sun goes down, it seems our guard also goes down with it, and we are more tempted than we are during the daytime.

Overeating and eating too late at night are the main reasons most people don't get enough sleep. The more a person eats, the more sleep he requires because more cleansing has to take place. So overeating makes it much more challenging to follow nature's time schedule. The best way to be successful with the Daylight Diet is to get to sleep early so you can wake early. If you awake too late in the day, your whole schedule will be off.

If you do not get the required amount of deep sleep, you will be tired and lazy, and you won't have the energy or excitement to achieve the divine eating schedule planned for you. Think about it:When we are excited about our life, we have no problem getting up early. Take, for example, a person on his or her wedding day. No matter what time they get to sleep the night before, they'll have no problem waking up extra early to start their busy and exciting day. They know there's a schedule that must be followed, and they do their best to be on time. We should all be just as excited and prepared every moment of our life to make sure a healthy planned schedule for us goes as smoothly as possible every day.

Going to bed at sundown or soon after means, then, that we should eat our last meal no later than the ninth hour of daylight (we will discuss that in another chapter), or at least five hours before going to bed. This guarantees that our meal has been digested and that our stomachs are empty enough to promote good, solid sleep.

When days are short

Days are short during the colder months, and, during the winter, the body is more stressed than it is during the warmer time of year. Wintertime foods are naturally denser in calories, and it takes more energy for our bodies to digest them. The increase in work and stress requires more rest and sleep. The nights are longer during these months, giving us a sign that we need to sleep more.

The foods of the warmer months are less dense, less caloric. They generally contain more liquid and digest more easily. The days are longer, and nights are shorter during these months, again giving us valuable clues for planning the ideal sleeping and eating schedules. Because of this, we require less sleep during the summer months.

Adjust your schedule accordingly: During the time of the year when days are shorter, eat your last meal earlier in the day, and go to bed earlier. When days are longer, you may eat later, and go to bed later, but do not eat when it's dark outside, and get to sleep at least several hours before midnight.

Likewise, you need to adjust your schedule if you live in parts of the world where the sun rarely sets. For instance, if you live in Alaska, it is light outside for most of summer. This doesn't mean you can eat all night or that there's no ideal time to go to sleep. The Daylight Diet is still the optimal health plan for you.

In these unique situations, there are other ways to tell the ideal digestion and sleeping times besides daylight and darkness. Under normal circumstances, the best digestion time starts at about the third hour of daylight, but when there is no normal sunrise and sunset, the body will be at its peak cleansing and rebuilding during the hours between 9 p.m. and 5 a.m., so these are the ideal times for sleeping. Peak digestion will be between

9 a.m. and 5 p.m., so these are the best hours for eating your meals. Even if you find yourself in these unique situations, you can adapt the Daylight Diet. As man continues to drift from his natural environment, it is still important to live according the divine schedule we were created to live by. I would suggest, in those situations, to pray about it first, but remember, no matter where you live, sleeping between the hours of 9 p.m. and 5 a.m. is usually the best way to go.

It is common these days for people to work a 9 a.m. to 5 p.m. job. It would be a healthy habit if people became accustomed to sleeping from 9 p.m. to 5 a.m.

Winding down

How else can we get good quality, deep sleep and ensure complete digestion and good health? Besides not eating late at night, relaxing or "winding down" before going to bed is always a good idea. Again, nature is the perfect model to learn from: Take, for instance, the sunrise. The transition from night to day doesn't happen immediately. There is an "adjustment" period from the first gleam of light along the horizon until the sun has completely risen. Sunset makes the opposite transition, but it is not immediate.

Like the sunrise and sunset, our bodies also need adjustment periods, between waking and getting on with our day, and between the day's activity and sleep. Too much stimulation will not allow us to relax enough to sleep, and then health problems can begin.

If the body has been stimulated right before bedtime—either by eating, watching television, sitting in a brightly lit room, playing a computer game, or even checking your email—it will be next to impossible to get to sleep at the intended time, and, as a result, difficult if not impossible to stay on the Daylight Diet. Remember: Once you start getting to bed late, you get into that rut of sleeping late in the morning and then getting to bed late the next night, too. Your digestive system doesn't get the chance to do its job, and health problems can begin.

About three hours before you intend to go to bed, stop working, turn off the television, dim the lights, and get off the computer. Go for a walk outside, listen to some classical music, or read the Scriptures and pray.

The best time to eat

Some people claim to be "morning people," while others say they are "night" people. The fact is, we are all day people. Other than nocturnal animals, most every other creature in nature gets up around sunrise. The birds start chirping, the flowers begin to open, and the air is the freshest it will be all day. Life truly seems to awaken all around as the sun comes up. Only the sick and diseased animals—and only sick and diseased people—will awaken well after sunrise.

You will certainly not be healthy if you are up all night and you sleep all day; staying up late at night goes against any health recommendations from anybody. People *choose* to be night people, and if you're one of them, you should know that you could *choose* to be a day person and get back on a healthful schedule. You will feel much better emotionally and physically. However, it may take a mental struggle to make the adjustment from enjoying the nightlife to the day life, but, in the long run, it will pay off.

Eating too soon after waking is not healthful, either, because it stimulates the body before you've had time to adjust naturally to the next phase of the day. If you get up at 7 or 8 a.m., you don't have enough time before starting work to adjust to daytime. This is another reason you should be waking up at 5 or 6 a.m. If you eat according to nature's timetable, you'll be able to give the body several hours to adjust before eating your first meal.

We must stick to nature's schedule to stay healthy. We should arise refreshed and ready to start our work at sunrise or even a few hours before. This may seem impossible to you now, but, all over the world, people who do usually live longer and enjoy better health.

Job circumstances

Special circumstances may cause some people to think they can't adopt the Daylight Diet—people who work nights, for instance, and have to sleep during the day.

All of us make choices about where and when we work, and if you value your health, you need to know that studies show that people who work the night shift are not as healthy as those who work in the daytime. That's why they call it the "graveyard" shift. Now I don't expect you to give up a job you love for a job you hate just because it's in the daytime, because enjoying your job is a large part of being healthy. The best answer, I think, is to find a job you love that has daytime hours. (And if you can't find one, make one.) It's the night owls who usually run into major issues with the Daylight Diet.

Liking what you do is important to your health. One of life's biggest stresses is feeling like an unhappy job situation controls your life. This leads people to overeat, to eat late at night, and to miss sleep. Take control of *your* life: Get a job you love, because even if you do work in the daytime, a job you hate will give you the same issues that will keep you from a healthful schedule of eating and sleeping.

How to Do It

The more you adhere to the Daylight Diet sleep schedule, the more practical and easier it will be to eat according to the plan He designed for your health. Likewise, the better you adhere to the set meal times, the easier it is to comply with the sleep schedule.

Unfortunately, many people are addicted to the way they do things and aren't willing to change their ways, even at the cost of their own health. They get themselves used to living an unhealthy lifestyle, and they cannot seem to leave their comfort zone: They don't want to change their diet. They don't want to stop watching television, and they don't want to exercise. They are addicted to a harmful lifestyle. They'd rather be sick and miss out on the health that could await them, than make the effort to change. My advice to people like this is:Try it before you deny it.

Rise each day early so you can start each day at the planned time. If you have a plan to get up at 6 a.m. to exercise, eat a nice breakfast at 8 a.m., and so on, but then you wake up late in the day, well, there goes your plan.

People today overwork and undersleep! A good sign of this is the need for an alarm clock to get out of bed, and the need for coffee or some other drug to stimulate the body once we are up. The amount of sleep each person needs is different for everyone based on their health, diet, age, and many other lifestyle factors. If you need coffee or an alarm clock, there is a good chance you are not getting enough sleep.

If sleep and rest are things we all love to do, why do we cut them short each morning? Many people will say it's because they have to get up and go to work. That is fine, but did you ever notice that when your work is your passion, you make sure you get enough rest to do a good job the next day? We get up with much energy and excitement to get the job done, but when we do not really like our job, we can barely get out of bed in the morning. The job we have can be a big factor in the amount of attention we put into our plan for getting enough rest. We all have a different lifestyle and different tasks to get done each day. We know how many hours we have each day to achieve our goals. Based on our needs, it is very helpful to plan our day wisely.

This book is about healthful eating, not sleep and rest, as it may seem; however; how much sleep we get can really make or break our attempts at the Daylight Diet.

With good effort, everyone can achieve excellent health by following the Daylight Diet. I suggest you proceed gradually to a point where you can comfortably eat less food. The best way to do that is, over a period of time, increase the quality of the food while reducing the amount. If you reduce the amount of food too quickly, you may cleanse too quickly, making things a little uncomfortable. If this is your experience, do not give up. Just slow down your cleanse by consuming a little more food.

The reason we cleanse once we reduce the amount of food is because our bodies have less digesting to do and can cleanse and detoxify. Skipping a meal or going on a fast actually assists the body in the cleansing. If someone who eats a lot of junk food and usually eats before bedtime goes a day with no food or just skips a meal, he will more than likely feel terrible and not sleep well because cleansing is taking place. But once his system has cleansed, and his body gets used to not eating later in the day, he will get the best sleep he has ever had.

CHAPTER 9

TWO MEALS A DAY

Everything you think you know about eating is wrong.

Eating whenever you have the urge is a theory I regret teaching, because there are too many factors that lead to impulsive eating. This philosophy usually leads to eating too much, too often, and too late. I have witnessed people destroying any health they had by this "listen to your body" concept.

The main reason for consuming food is nourishment, but today one of the primary factors that bring about the desire for food is emotion. This is where we get the phrase "emotional eating." As I travel all over the world, I often observe people desire food not based on their need for nourishment, but because it appears enticing to them. There is a popular old joke that goes like this: I'm on a seafood diet. When I see food, I eat it. Marketers know this, too, and they play on it; we think we are hungry, but they have just fooled us. For these reasons, I no longer suggest we eat when we "feel" hungry. Instead, it's wise to eat at the same time every day.

Plan, plan, plan.

Do your best to have the meals the same time each day but not too often. A common eating pattern of breakfast, brunch, lunch, and dinner, plus many snacks in between has become common nowadays but is too much food. One of the worst recommendations about diet these days is to eat many small meals throughout the day. This is a harmful practice, because it never gives the organs a chance to fully digest the last meal and rest. It also greatly contributes toward overeating, because, once in the habit of eating often, it's too challenging to eat less often.

A lifetime of eating at different times every day often results in digestive problems at a much earlier age than people who eat at the same times each day. When meals are not planned ahead, emotions and habits usually control our food desires and cause us to eat when we're not really hungry.

It starts in childhood

Newborn babies need to feed often — their stomachs are tiny and empty quickly and often. The good thing is they get full very quickly and rarely eat too much. Once they are full, they are done! However the older the baby becomes, the less often the feeding times should be. Older babies and young children who eat as often as a newborn would be overfed and, unlike newborn babies, don't always stop eating once they are full.A common pattern I see today among young parents also encourages overfeeding:They feed their babies whenever they cry, often using food as a comfort. This practice of using food as a means of comfort usually carries over to the child and grownup years and may result in adults who eat to comfort themselves rather than fill their stomachs.

Cravings versus hunger

When people get a craving, they think it's because the body needs that food; that's why they are experiencing the craving. At first, this can seem to make sense, but once I see the low-quality, junk food a person is craving, I know it's really not a nutritional need that creates that craving. It's usually some form of emotional eating, not true hunger.

The best way to be successful at the Daylight Diet is to establish meal times and stick to them. You must understand and establish control over your cravings. You must also understand what causes the feeling of true hunger. In 1870, Dr. Dio Lewis explained what causes the feeling of hunger:

"It was thought for a long time that the sensation of hunger was produced by the gastric juice attacking the coats of the empty stomach. When food was present, the stomach juice was busy with that; but when the food had passed on and left the stomach empty, the powerful solvent attacked the stomach itself. It was thought that this produced the gnawing of hunger. But when it was found out that not a drop of this gastric juice was furnished while the stomach was empty, that theory was abandoned.

"Dr. Beaumont, who enjoyed the rarest opportunities to study the functions of the stomach, suggested that the feeling of hunger was probably owing to a distended state of the vessels which furnish the gastric juice. And he thought this view was greatly strengthened by the prodigious rapidity with which the juice is poured in upon the first introduction of food, showing, as he argues, that the juice was already existing and waiting in the vessels or follicles that furnish it.

"Again, physiologists have thought the feeling of hunger was caused by the two sides of the empty stomach rubbing against each other. But these and various other explanations which have reference to the condition of the stomach along fail to recognize the systemic want which is the real cause of hunger."

"Let me illustrate. I have eaten but two meals a day for many years, one at half past seven a.m., the other at one o'clock p.m. Between my dinner (the noon time meal in 1870 was called dinner) and the next morning's breakfast is eighteen hours. During twelve of these, I presume, the stomach is mostly empty; but I never feel the sensation of hunger. I have induced hundreds to live in the same way, and, after a few days, not one of them feels the sensation of hunger.

"A gentleman, now prominent in the field of health reform, was in my service some years ago as a teacher of gymnastics. He worked very hard and evinced remarkable endurance. Now, when I state that he ate but one meal a day and never suffered from hunger, it will be seen that the above theories fail to explain the sensation under consideration. The stomach must have been empty eighteen to twenty hours out of every twenty-four; but, notwithstanding this emptiness, the gastric juice did not gnaw the lining coats, the vessels were not painfully distended, nor did the coats of the stomach rub against each other, producing the discomfort of hunger.

"A man is hungry all over, his legs not less than his stomach. The feeling in his legs is restlessness, but the stomach is endowed with a peculiar sensibility, so that hunger in that organ is a faintness and gnawing. The hunger is not dependent in the least upon the emptiness of the stomach. For example, a man is convalescent from a fever. He has lost thirty pounds. The demand for nutriment is urgent. This man may fill his stomach with baker's bread and potatoes; his hunger is not appeased, for, although his stomach is distended, the systemic want is not met, and his appetite continues.

"A striking illustration of this dependence of the local upon the general is found in thirst, which is felt mostly in the throat. If a tube be carefully introduced through a dog's side into the stomach, and the dog, when very thirsty, be allowed to thrust his head into a tub of water, he will go on drinking for an hour, stopping only a moment to rest and take breath. The throat is flooded; but, as the feeling of thirst is dependent on a want of the system, and the water running out of the stomach through the tube fails to satisfy this want of the system, so the thirst continues, though the animal may have swallowed gallons. But, if we inject a quantity of water into a vein of the leg of this thirsty dog, the feeling of thirst in his throat, though it has not been touched by a drop of water, will speedily disappear.

"Bernard made an opening into the oesophagus of a horse, tied the lower portion, and then allowed the animal to drink. He drunk an immense quantity, but the water not passing into his stomach, the thirst was unquenched.

"Dr. Gairdner, of Edinburgh, reports an interesting case, that of a man whose throat had been cut and the oesophagus divided. The thirst, in this case, was insatiable, though many gallons of water were drunk in a day; but when a little water was injected into the stomach, the sensation was soon relieved."

No matter how many meals you eat, it's best to stick to a pattern and eat at the same times every day. Among the laws of health and digestion, this one of regularity is preeminently important.

How many meals each day

> *I advise but two meals a day. There can be no doubt that two meals a day are better than three. I have no doubt that the two-meal system is likewise better for working men.* — **Dr. Dio Lewis**

Nowadays, the average person eats too often. There is no doubt in my mind if people cut down on the number of meals they eat and the amount of food in those meals, the rates of disease would greatly be reduced.

We should all strive for a two-meals-a-day system—three meals at most, but never more than three and no snacking in between meals. This is the only way we can assure we are giving ourselves all the needed ingredients to achieve the Daylight Diet on a regular basis. The highest level of the Daylight Diet is not eating at nighttime, but also, at least four to six hours between each meal, resting before and after each meal, and not eating within five hours of going to bed for the night. How can we have time to do all of these things if we are eating more than two times a day? That's the point: We can't!

If you eat three times a day, you can adjust your schedule so you have a little less time between meals and a little less time before going to sleep. However, if you eat more than three times a day, you will not reap all of the health benefits of the Daylight Diet. (A practical plan for achieving the Daylight Diet is outlined in Chapter 19. It is important to get a good understanding of everything before attempting the program, so please read this whole book before moving ahead.)

As a first step to break the addiction to eating at night—and something everyone can start doing right now—is to eat as much as you want in the daytime, but get out of the habit of eating after the sun goes down, or after 6 p.m., whichever comes first. The sun stays up in the summer time months often until late in the evening, but one of the essential keys of the Daylight Diet is not to eat late at night regardless of whether it is light outside or not.

Eating many meals throughout the day and stopping at night-time is better than continuing to eat late at night, but it is still not ideal. We need to train ourselves to eat less often, just as we trained ourselves to eat more often.

All stages of the Daylight Diet are only going to work if we have a healthy sleep schedule; this means getting to bed before midnight (the more hours before the better) and rising with the sun, or before the sun comes up, if you had enough hours of sleep. If you are going to sleep later and wake up later, the Daylight Diet will be much harder to achieve.

Extra food slows you down.

As the body becomes more efficient, you will do better with less food. Extra food is very stimulating. When you finally get healthy, you won't need that stimulation. The problem with stimulation is that there is always a crash; then you need more food to get that feeling again.

People today worry too much about counting calories or keeping their metabolism high, but high calories and fast metabolism speed up the aging process—they do not reduce it. What reduces the aging process is temperance in eating. Studies prove a restricted calorie diet is best.

I am very active on a two-meals-a-day system. I've finished 100-mile bike rides and felt fine. Professor Arnold Ehret, author of *The Mucusless Diet Healing System* and other great books, gives great examples in his book of how active and strong a person can be with less food if they are clean inside. Ehret conducted many long-term fasting experiments—some more than 50 days—and would then go on long hikes and engage in strengthening exercises just to prove that, if done with wisdom, people can have more energy, strength, and endurance, eating far less than they are used to.

According to Ehret, the human body is like a complex plumbing system of blood vessels, driven by the air of the lungs, with the blood-fluid constantly moving, all regulated by the heart. Proper breathing, clean air, and non-mucus foods will keep our pipes clean and help the body work properly for an incredibly long time without tiring. But no matter what we do, if we consistently overeat, we will always tire quickly.

All the health writers I showcase in this book agree we need very little food if we're eating the right amounts at the right times. Unlike the common thinking today that we need food for fuel, food does not give us energy; it only temporarily stimulates us. When our body is clean and free of mucus, slime, obstruction, toxins, or whatever you want to call it, you can thrive on very little.

Many people today eat much more than the Daylight Diet suggests and actually feel great (because of the stimulation provided by the food). But I warn you: This will catch up with you if you keep abusing your body. I should know: I learned the hard way. Some people may get away with this overindulgence longer than others, but just because you have gotten away with it, it is not an excuse to keep doing it. Once you find out the truth— that all that extra food is creating wear and tear inside your body—it's wise to stop. Our amazing bodies are a gift, but the real gift is that we have time to understand our harmful ways and change them. Doing the same things over and over and expecting different results is the definition of "insanity."

Raw food author and nutritionist Dr. Fred Bisci has been eating only two meals a day for more than 40 years. He explains why the concept of eating many meals throughout the day is mistakenly believed to be right but it is not:

First, Bisci says, people snack to maintain their blood sugar levels, but this is only somewhat valid if your diet is high in carbohydrates and creates insulin spikes followed by low blood sugar, in which case it is advisable to raise them again. But, Dr. Bisci asks, why correct a "wrong" with a "wrong?" The healthful choice is to turn the first "wrong" into a "right" and to establish an eating style that maintains blood sugar levels between meals *without* snacking.

Second, snacking leads to food fermentation in the digestive tract, because the previous snack, still only partially digested, impedes the progress of the food following it.

Third, and most harmful, eating too often prevents the body from going through a detoxification process, which it must do on a daily basis if a person is to live a long and healthy life. By eating too many meals a day, you never give your stomach a chance to empty, and your body is unable to detoxify and keep you clean on a cellular level.

Dr. Stanley Bass, another longtime health author, is in his 90s. He claims one of the secrets to his advanced age is frugal eating: For years, he lived on one meal a day. I also know a man, 108 years old, who is in excellent shape; he claims the key to his great health is eating very little.

What about active people? Are two meals a day enough? Dr. Lewis writes:

> "I knew a number of carpenters who tried the two-meal system, eating nothing after one o'clock, taking at supper time a cup of milk and hot tea, and retiring early. Most of them were not only satisfied, but were enthusiastic over their clear heads and nimble muscles."

According to Professor Ehret, getting tired is the result of three factors, all related to overeating:

- A reduction in strength due to excessive digestion
- The congestion and "heating up" of blood vessels, which causes dilation
- Activity-induced mucus excretion, which causes tox-

ins to be secreted, resulting in "self-poisoning" and "rebound-poisoning"

According to Ehret, oxygen is what we need to achieve energy—not food—because it is the basic element for build-up, repair, and replacement. Food creates an internal environment that prevents oxygen from doing its job—just the opposite of what most people believe it does. (This explains why my IBD started to heal, and I actually gained weight during my three-day fast when my disease would worsen every time I ate.)

Nothing takes more energy from the body than digestion of food. The more you eat, the more stimulation you will need to deal with the lack of energy that results from the digestion. How many times have you had to have a nap after a big Thanksgiving dinner? Or could hardly stay awake and sometimes even fall asleep at the table after eating a big meal? The reason is because too much food uses massive energy to digest. Yet, if clean and healthy, the body needs very little food, but it can still perform much physical activity. I have even seen people eat a small amount of fruit and have enough energy to run a marathon. Even the hardest workers these days don't come close to the extremes a marathon puts on the body, but they still often believe they must "eat for energy." This may be somewhat true for an unhealthy person because when they consume less, the cleansing process may make them feel weak; but once clean and healthy, we will all thrive on very little as long as it's good quality.

Ehret was a brilliant man, not only because he understood the human body and about health and diet, but also because he refused to listen to ignorant and uninformed people talking about their "daily necessity and natural urge to eat a lot." He often said these people talk but have never experienced how easy and long one can work or walk without tiring in a lifestyle that includes fasting and a fruit diet.

We should be very active and enjoy life. If we are active, we can consume more food within our two or even three meals a day, but no hard-working man or woman needs to eat more than two or three times a day at most, as long as it is done wisely. It is always advisable to eat less rather than more.

Ideal eating times

Eating late at night is the most common dietary problem. Eating the wrong foods, eating too often, and eating too much are other widespread issues, but late-night eating is the most serious.

The routine of eating three meals a day or more lasting well into the night has become a popular trend only in the last 150 years. There is no real wisdom behind this practice and surely no health advantage. Even experts and health writers who have never studied the topic agree the body is more efficient at digestion when the sun is shining and that going to sleep on a full stomach is not a healthy practice.

As I discussed earlier in this chapter, it is best to have the same mealtimes each day, but that does not necessarily mean eating at the same time each day, at least, not by a man-made clock (another unhealthful, new custom of man, telling time by a man-made clock instead of the sun and moon). The time of the sunrise and of the sunset changes each day, so 6 a.m. today on a man-made clock is not the exact time as 6 a.m. tomorrow. The "natural" day has a different length each day. The man-made clock never takes this into consideration, and this is where the major confusion happens. (This is also a topic no one writes about or discusses, yet is so vital to good health.)

When it comes to sleeping times and mealtimes, what you need to do is ignore the time on the man-made clock. Your goal is to eat at the same time each day, and, regardless of what the man-made clock shows, the only way to figure out the same time each day is to start counting from sunrise.

Flora and fauna

Every natural rhythm calculates time by the sun and moon. Plants, ocean waves, and even animals live their entire lives according to the sun and moon. Plants open and close their flowers at the same times each day. No matter how much we may talk to animals or plants and tell them what to do, they have coded within them only one way to respond, and that is with their natural instincts. Their behavior patterns may change times based on seasonal or climate changes, but as long as they're in their natural environments, they will respond to nature's cycles.

However, if you take plants or animals out of their natural environment without mimicking it, they will die. For them to have any chance of survival, you would have to continuously supply them with what they receive naturally. The first (and last) sign that something is wrong is they are no longer on their natural schedule. If you can find a way to move a plant or animal to another environment but keep its natural schedule, it will survive, but it will not thrive as it would in its natural environment. The longer you keep the plant away from its natural environment, the less quality of life it will produce.

Florists do a good job imitating plants' original environment. Zookeepers create wonderful environments for animals that are native to far-flung regions of the world. Just buying a goldfish and keeping it in a fish tank in your home is a decent job at creating a similar environment for the animals. Man can find ways to mimic the sunlight and the rain by way of fluorescent lights and water to keep plants on their correct schedule; we will cut and build a forested area for animals, or spend time and money on a beautiful fish tank to duplicate the beauty of the ocean floor, but we cannot manage to keep our own body on its correct natural schedule. We certainly have the capability to do it; most people just choose not to.

The tide rushes in.

To figure out the best times for us to eat and how often we should eat, we can look to yet another force of nature: tides. These tides of nature work in harmony with our own body rhythms and reveal the ideal times for sleeping, eating, cleansing, and being active. The farther we stray from these times, the more stress we put on our body to stay healthy. Just as a plant will survive in a mimicked environment on a different schedule, so can we, thanks to the amazing power built within us. We have an amazing power to adapt, but every time we do, something happens that makes us sick and shortens our life in the process.

Today, everyone is looking to be healthy and live a long life, and they're spending lots of time and money trying to do it. From growing sprouts for years, I have learned there is a science to getting the freshest, biggest, tastiest, and most nutritious sprouts. There are several factors that contribute to my green thumb, but my basic practice is to keep them on a schedule.

Eating anytime during the day is much better than consuming food at nighttime, but the best time to eat is when the body is naturally in its digestion rhythm. From my study of the Bible and many other health books, I have concluded there are two times a day when the digestive system hits its peak: the third hour and the ninth hour of daylight.

Eating the third and ninth hour of daylight may seem unusual because they're not the customary eating times we are used to. (And we are not in the habit of telling time by the sunrise and sunset.) Plus, it is only two times a day as opposed to the traditional three meals per day. But, as we've discussed before, as long as the quality of the food is very high, two meals a day should be sufficient for our nutritional needs.

Now you can begin to understand why getting to bed and rising at the correct times are so vital to our health. Your first meal should be taken at the third hour after sunrise. If you've slept past sunrise, you've thrown off your entire schedule.

The third and ninth hours

According to the man-made clock, the third hour after sunrise usually starts somewhere between 7 a.m. and 9 a.m. for our first meal, and the ninth hour between 2 p.m. and 4 p.m. for our second meal. Because nature calculates time by a different method, you are really not eating at a different phase of the day, because no matter what the man-made clock says, you will always be eating at the third and ninth hours of daylight.

The correct, specific time for your two meals, of course, will always depend on the season and the time of sunrise where you live. It may still be light out at 7 a.m. in the summer but dark at 7 a.m. in the winter where you live, and it's never good to eat when it's dark outside; wait three hours after sunrise, no matter what the season or where you happen to be, and you will be eating your first meal at the optimal time.

There is a helpful website where you can just input the times of sunset and sunrise where you are, and it will tell you the times of the third and ninth hour: www.the-branch.org. (You can also download a spreadsheet from that website that will help you figure out the times each day.) In case you are not able to get online every day, here is how to figure it out:

There are 12 hours in the daytime and 12 hours in the night. However, we must not assume there are 60 minutes always in an hour. That is a man-made idea. Only on the equator is the length of day hours the same as night hours. The times of the sunrise and sunset determine how long an hour truly is. Along the equator, there are equal amounts of daylight and darkness, but anywhere else in the world, that is always changing. In the winter, there are more hours of darkness, and in the summer, more light. So how do you tell what the true third hour and ninth hour are?

Find out from a calendar, a weather website, a newspaper, or the Farmer's Almanac the times of sunrise and sunset. Once you have those times, the rest is easy to figure out. Here's an example:

- Suppose sunrise is 6 a.m. and sunset is 6 p.m. The third hour of daylight would start at 8 a.m., and the ninth hour would begin at 2 p.m.

- Now, for a more complicated example, suppose sunrise was 6:33 a.m. and sunset, 8:17 p.m.:
- 12 hours = 720 minutes (if there were 60 minutes to the hour)
- Add any "extra" minutes, in other words, any minutes exceeding 720 minutes: From 6:33 a.m. to 8:17 p.m. is 13 hours, 47 minutes, or 104 extra minutes.
- Add 720 + 104 = 824 minutes
- Divide 824 by 12 to get the "true" total minutes in an hour, 68 minutes (in this example)
- Starting from the time of sunrise, use 68 minutes for each hour to calculate the beginning of the third and ninth hours, as in this example:
- 6:33 a.m. + 68 + 68 = 8:49 a.m., which is the beginning of the third hour
- 6:33 a.m.+ 68 + 68 + 68 + 68 + 68 + 68 + 68 + 68= 3:37 p.m., the beginning of the ninth hour
- (If you choose to eat 3 meals a day, eat the first a little earlier and the last meal a little later, and add one meal in the middle.)

Getting started.

Getting started on the Daylight Diet eating plan of two meals a day at the third and ninth hours doesn't have to be difficult. Here are some easy steps you can take in the beginning to familiarize yourself with eating at the right times:

- Do not eat when it is dark outside, or do not eat after a certain time, such as 6 p.m.
- If you did not figure the exact times of the third and ninth hours, just try eating around 8:30 a.m. and 2:30 p.m. that day.

- If eating at those times is too hard, try to eat just two (or three if you must, but no more than three) meals a day, but not within an hour of waking or within five hours of going to sleep. Your last meal of the day should be no later than 6 p.m., but the earlier, the better.
- Never eat when it is dark outside. In the wintertime, when days are shorter, your last meal may be at 3 or 4 p.m.
- If you have a nighttime job, consider the impact this has on your health. If you cannot change to a daytime job, then eat as much as you can when it is daylight outside so you are not hungry at nighttime, and try not to eat during the middle of the night.

We are all different.

Each person is in a different situation, and the condition, of our body is never identical to anyone else's, so we have to pay attention and give our own body the attention it needs. We can't base this on what everyone else is doing, but on what our body requires. We have all been created to live according to the same divine schedule. No matter our situation, the plan does not adjust to our situation; we have to alter our circumstances to fit the divine plan for our life.

No matter how different the stages of our health may be, there is a universal, ideal time to consume our food. Just like every rhythm of life, the time never changes based on how we feel or daylight saving time (another harmful man-made custom). The immortal times never change.

However, the conditions of our bodies are at different stages, based on how we've treated them. Our vitality, or lack of it, determines the exact type of diet we need. A person sick and lacking nutrients will need a much different food plan than a healthy person who has been eating a good diet for many years. No matter what the state of our bodies and the history of our diets, we all deserve the best quality food for our particular situations. We will talk more about the quality of food later, but keep in mind the best times to eat those foods are the same for everyone.

Even though we have all been designed to keep the same eating and sleeping pattern for ideal health, during our daily lives we each have different chores and jobs each day. For some of us, switching our eating and sleeping patterns will be simple because we have a lot of free time to do so. For others, it may not be as easy due to our hectic lifestyle. For instance, a single person with no job will have a much easier time than a big family where both parents are working. Sometimes our jobs may not coincide with the requirements of the Daylight Diet, but that is not an excuse *not* to make an effort.

It takes time to adjust, and, depending on our situations, some of us will adjust sooner than others. Decide for yourself what is truly feasible or what you're just doing out of habit. For instance, if your family is in the habit of eating dinner around 8 p.m. every night, that's not a healthy habit; however, if everyone is working until 7 p.m., it may not be feasible to eat together before 8 p.m. This does not make it wise to completely give up on the idea, however. Not following the Daylight Diet just because you have a good excuse does not eliminate the potential damage that results when you're not following a natural schedule. Instead of the family eating together for dinner at 8 p.m., maybe they can have their first meal of the day together.

I do not expect all of you to be able to switch your schedules and turn your habits instantly. Some of you may never decide to change, but we can all make some adjustments that help. Perhaps you'll no longer eat anything after dinner. Or maybe you'll go for a walk in the morning before you eat breakfast. It's very important that we evaluate our own situations, but even more important to remember that, like a plant, we are designed to live according to a divine schedule if we want to thrive in our environment.

CHAPTER 10

ADRENAL FATIGUE

How TV, sugar, caffeine, and computers are making you sick

We live in a world full of constant stress, and when we do not deal with it wisely, we overeat and eat late at night. In addition to worry and fear, people today are overworked and do not get enough rest. Add to this the quick-paced business world of emails, phone calls, text messages, and Blackberries, and it builds even more stress. Financial pressures, personality conflicts, reliance on stimulants like caffeine and sugar, digestive problems, too much exercise, illness or infection, and unresolved emotional issues lead us to a breaking point. No matter what you call it, we are burning ourselves out.

During this burnout stage, we may sometimes feel OK because it stimulates us. We may *feel* energized, but too much stimulation is a form of stress, even if we perceive stimulation as a good thing at the time. Other than food, many other things stimulate us emotionally and mentally: music, video games, television, worries, danger, high noise levels, and even bright lights. We even have to be careful about things such as exercise because, even though good for us, too much is perceived by our bodies as a stressor.

When we are under stress, our bodies release a hormone called *adrenaline*, which is a built-in mechanism that boosts all of our senses to react more quickly. An example is when we hear a balloon pop. It may make the same loud noise as a gunshot, but we clearly know the difference. The problem is, our body doesn't know the difference, and any loud noise noise is going to boost our adrenaline.

Every stress creates a demand on the body and on the adrenal glands in particular. If we are under stress all the time because of all the stimulation taking place, our adrenal glands just keep pumping out the adrenaline. The result is adrenal glands that are constantly on high alert. This can exhaust the adrenal glands—a serious issue, because your adrenal glands produce a variety of hormones that are essential to life. The effects of adrenal exhaustion can be detrimental to our health.

Fatigue and weakness are usually the first signs of adrenal fatigue. This is important to understand, because it means our bodies will become unable to fight off disease. If not dealt with, all this stress can lead to many other issues that are so common today, such as, muscle and bone loss, depression, hormonal imbalance, and eventually even cancer. These are just a few of the many issues caused as a result of getting "stressed out." There is a strong connection with adrenal fatigue and emotional eating, and both usually result in late-night binge eating.

To be healthy, we need to support the immune system and not add stress to it. Once we stress our nervous system, we start burning nutrients in excess. This will lead to deficiencies, depression, and, yes, insomnia. Then the door will be open to many other issues, such as adrenal fatigue.

These days, we engage in too many activities that produce adrenaline rush, including even too many fitness exercises, or working out too often, bungee jumping, and other extreme sports all may seem like fun at the time, but they are making the adrenal glands work more often than they were ever meant to.

Of all those activities, eating at nighttime is the most harmful, because nothing stimulates and exhausts the body more than eating. A dance ends, TV shows are over, sports don't last too long, but well after a person has eaten, the body stays stimulated, doing its work, even when we try to rest.

This may not seem too serious to us because everyone else seems to be stressed out in some form, too, thanks to the common, fast-paced lives people are living today; but that doesn't make it OK. If the stresses aren't dealt with, and if the exhausting and stressful lifestyle continues, adrenal exhaustion can lead to conditions that can be fatal.

To sleep, perchance to cleanse

So many people complain they have a hard time falling asleep at night. Instead of trying to find a way to relax, they do just the opposite: They turn on the TV or the computer or some other stimulating activity, such as eating.

Watching television or using the computer right before bed will almost guarantee that you won't get to sleep. Why? Because they are stimulants. I notice it takes me two to three hours to overcome the stimulating effects of television and computers before I can sleep. According to the Daylight Diet, you need to be in bed several hours before midnight to get a good night's sleep and give the body a chance to do its work. If it takes you a couple of hours to come down after watching TV or playing on the computer and you don't get to bed before about 9 p.m., well, you do the math. You're going to be awake when your body needs you to sleep.

The other thing insomniacs do, of course, is eat. But food is a stimulant, too, and will not help you go back to sleep, although you may wonder how food can be so stimulating if we feel so drowsy after a big meal? Here's how:

Eating takes its toll on the body. Every bite of food you put in your body takes a massive amount of work to digest. Every part of the body is put into action one way or another to deal with the food you eat. Even before food enters the body, the thought of eating and even the smell of the food alert the organs to produce enzymes and other digestive juices in preparation for the food. Once the food has entered the digestive system, the process moves into high gear. If you do not overindulge, you may feel energized from food because of the stimulating affect, particularly if we've eaten a food such as sugar or caffeine. But if we overeat, the body has to work so hard to digest the food that it loses more energy than it appears to be receiving. The same thing happens when we eat food in poor combinations, eat low quality food or eat too late at night.

There is a difference between energy and stimulation. Energy is the result we get when we eat a good diet, get the proper amount of rest, and live a healthful lifestyle. Stimulation is something that makes us feel a spark of energy—but that's a false energy, in a way. Real energy or a sense of well-being is another form of vitality or health, while stimulation, if not just the needed amount, is unhealthful, and stress forming.

Sugar and caffeine

People who eat junk food rely on stimulating foods to make up for the lack of energy they feel. That means they rely mostly on sugar, caffeine, and artificial additives to make them feel awake and aware. This is especially true of people who eat at night.

We know processed sugars and caffeine are not good for us, but we also have to remember that even the naturally occurring sugars and caffeine don't do us any favors if we eat too much of them.

Too much sugar causes insulin to be put into the blood at a quicker rate than it should be. This spike in insulin puts tremendous stress on the pancreas. Too much sugar in the diet is always going to result in health problems one way or another. At the very least, it saps nutrients from the body, makes you feel tired, and puts on pounds because it is so high in calories. At the worst, it can result in hypoglycemia, which, if not addressed, can eventually become type 2 diabetes. Too much sugar also supports cancer growth in the body.

It is no mystery to me that sugar and caffeine cause so many health problems today. I truly believe that, if people didn't eat when it was dark outside, they wouldn't have to rely on these harmful foods, because they wouldn't feel the need to be stimulated or energized. But people have developed a lifestyle of living off the adrenaline rush, and sugar and caffeine help bring them back up when they crash. Add lack of sleep, emotional stimulation from television, movies, and video games, plus pushing themselves with too much physical exercise and working overtime, and you quickly see more and more people suffering from adrenal fatigue.

Unfortunately, even people who are eating healthfully seem to be getting burned out. I find many people suffer from impaired function, ranging from significant adrenal stress to complete adrenal exhaustion, or adrenal burnout. The one factor most people have in common who suffer from adrenal fatigue is that they eat at nighttime.

Night eating syndrome

There is a condition called night eating syndrome (NES), in which people develop insomnia and believe they can't sleep unless they eat something; food helps them go to sleep. Some people with this condition won't even remember in the morning that they ate before they went to bed, even when they binge, which is not uncommon. Some even wake up three and four times a night to snack some more.

What's interesting to me about NES is that it was around 1955 that television was becoming an important part of the American lifestyle. For years since then, experts have made connections between the stimulation of television and overeating. I think you could add another connection: the stimulation of television prevents you from getting a good night's sleep.

Watching too much television can lead to depression, lack of sleep, and obesity. I just picture people falling asleep with the TV on, the remote control in one hand and food in the other. They may wake periodically to take a bite, or during every commercial break they are running to the fridge for some high-carb, high-sugar snack like cake or cookies. It's just a matter of time before doctors name the new disorder TMTVS, or Too Much TV Syndrome.

Just say no to TV.

Technology is making our life so simple, right? Wrong. It is making us lazy and is keeping us more occupied than ever before. Television, email, cell phones, computers—people just don't have time to think. They're so busy *reacting* to technology and following the crowd. They can't find the time to eat during the day, so they feed their hunger habit late at night.

The biggest hurdle most people have to overcome to succeed at The Daylight Diet is television. There's almost nothing that saps more of our time and energy than the boob tube. More than anything else, it is television that keeps us up at night and keeps us eating when we shouldn't. Advertisers understand how people think, and they know how to make us hungry when we aren't.

We've already discussed how important it is to eat the right foods, in the right amounts, at the right times. Nighttime is not the right time, but people have lost all sense of time and natural scheduling because they schedule their entire lives around their favorite shows on television. Cable TV and the networks have become our new clocks. The television networks call it "programming" for a reason: They're programming you to be on their schedule. We live during a time now where people spend more hours than ever before watching television. We also live during a time when there is more disease than ever before. See the connection?

Just the name—"tell-a-vision"—should make us see it for what it is: a box that tells us about visions. The mind control through scientific machinery and human mind-manipulation being told today on the tell-a-vision is not a healthful message. I would say 90 percent of the shows on television today consist of messages that program us to live against our natural schedule. Not only do we attempt to enjoy these messages, but we also allow our children to experience these harmful images. What the eyes absorb can easily become part of our life; it brainwashes us. And the whole experience makes us physically lazy.

I suggest you get rid of your television, if you haven't already. Or keep the machine, and watch only quality programs and movies; control what you watch and when you watch it. The quality of your life will improve. You will start responding to nature's schedule for your body. You will go to sleep earlier, wake earlier, and eat better. And you'll be able to easily adopt the Daylight Diet.

Adrenal fatigue can almost always be relieved with some adjustment in diet and lifestyle, but I have found the quickest way to turn the issue around is the Daylight Diet.

The need for stimulation to stay awake or focused is just another reason why eating only two times a day is more healthful than three or more. When the body is not burdened with the job of consistently digesting and detoxing from food, a person will have more true energy and won't need to rely on stimulants to stay awake or focused. The cleaner the body, the clearer the mind. It all works together.

PART 3

Preparing Yourself to Eat Less Food, Less Often

CHAPTER 11

UNDERSTANDING NIGHTTIME HUNGER

Maybe we need better food.

People eat at nighttime for a lot of reasons: boredom, conditioning, habit, false sense of hunger, taste, and emotional emptiness. But I think an even more common reason is that they are not giving their bodies the nutrients they need during the daytime so they can feel satiated by nighttime. Another thing to remember is that the body has to work harder to digest food at night than it does during the daytime—even if the food you eat at night is high quality.

Much of the food available today has too few nutrients, so no matter how much people stuff themselves throughout the day, they will always desire more food at night since they're not meeting their nutritional needs. Think about fast food: A hamburger and fries from the drive-through will certainly fill you up, and because it is so caloric, it should probably fill you up for an entire day. But it leaves us dissatisfied because it lacks nutrients and, an hour or so later, we're eating again, to satisfy our nutrient needs.

Too much isn't the answer.

Dr. Dio Lewis talked about big eaters in his books. He wrote about a man who ate four times a day, thinking he needed that much food to support his physical endurance because he had a very active job. He came to Dr. Lewis complaining his stomach wasn't well. When he told Dr. Lewis he ate four times a day, Dr. Lewis told him his problem was that he ate like a pig; that is why he was suffering with stomach issues. The man told Dr. Lewis that, even though he eats four meals a day, he is often faint, and that he needed an extra meal to keep up his strength.

Dr. Lewis explained physiology to him in great detail and finally convinced him to eat only two small meals a day: the first at 7 a.m. and the other around noon. Then, Dr. Lewis told him, get to bed early every night.

Within 15 days, the man was no longer faint, and he was rapidly recovering. Eventually, he became very healthy and active again. Of course, this man quickly became a strong advocate of eating just two moderate meals a day.

If the food you're eating is high quality—raw, fresh, organic fruits, vegetables, nuts, and seeds—and if you are eating at the ideal times, you will hardly ever feel hungry, particularly at nighttime. Here is what Dr. Lewis says in his book about temperate eating, energy, hunger, and eating just two meals a day.

"Temperate people, with healthy stomachs, never feel their stomachs, forget they have stomachs: while these enormous eaters are always hungry, or faint, or bloated, or troubled with eructation's, or acidity, or diarrhea, or some other condition, showing a morbid and unhappy state of the digestive apparatus.

"Nearly all the very strong men, and all the very active men with whom I have been acquainted, have been moderate eaters. The physiology of these remarkable facts is simply this: It takes a large amount of nerve force to digest food. With these prodigious eaters, all the nerve force is in the stomach, and so nothing is left for brain or muscle.

"Persons having a good stomach to begin with, can, by long practice, learn to digest an enormous quantity of food. If they give their whole force and vitality to this business of grinding grists, they can, in the course of even a short life, grind through immense quantities. But as a steady and regular and only occupation, it is hardly consonant with the loftiest ambition, and so I advise the other policy, pursued by such as have nobler aims and purposes in life. That other policy is to find out just how much food is needed to run the machine, exactly what fuel is best to keep the steam at the best working point, and then never pass these bounds.

"I was astonished at the results of an experiment upon my own person. For years I had eaten three hearty meals a day. At length, upon a careful consideration of the physiology of digestion, I found I was probably using too much of my force in that function. I reduced to two meals a day, and to about one-half, altogether, of the quantity of food I had been using. I can't tell you what a freedom in mental and bodily activity I experienced. I know scores of men with large heads, and fine, vigorous bodies, who consume so much of their nerve force in digestion that they have nothing left with which to achieve those grand triumphs which, otherwise, would be so easy to them."

It all comes down to this: If we can physically and mentally satisfy ourselves on two small meals a day at the right times, we will not get a craving to eat at nighttime. We get the feeling of hunger when we do not satisfy our body's nutritional needs.

Habit versus hunger

There is a difference between habit hunger and real starvation. If you let your body go hungry long, and it truly needs nourishment, eventually it can lead to starvation. As long as the correct nourishment is given to the body, and the body is working correctly to assimilate those nutrients, starvation would be almost impossible. Like Dr. Lewis's patient above, most people don't understand that they don't need a lot of food to satisfy their hunger; they think, "the more, the better." This is what most of us learned as kids growing up, and it is often the only way we know how to get rid of the sensation of hunger. But we never stop to think that, if eating is truly the cure for hunger, why are we always eating? Wouldn't the food we eat take care of the issue?

It's what we eat, not how much.

Like the thirsty dog back in Chapter 9, whose thirst was not quenched until its leg was injected with water, we will keep eating until our body has obtained all the nutrients it needs. What's important is not how much we eat or drink, but how much of it our body will be able to use that determines how often we get hungry. When we consume high quality food during the daytime, we will not feel hungry at nighttime. We don't even need a lot of food during the day, just enough to meet our needs. We all have different nutritional needs, based on many variables. No two people will require the same amount, but the key is to reach the amount that satisfies us.

People tend to consume much more food than they need to these days, and it doesn't seem to matter why they are hungry. Whether your feeling of hunger is brought on by habit or emotions, the bottom line is there is a trend today to consume much more food than we need to. No matter how much food you consume, if it is low quality, you will not give the body what it needs, and it will crave more food—not because it needs food, but because it needs nutrients that it should be getting from the foods.

When the body doesn't waste energy by trying to metabolize the wrong foods at the wrong time, or by having to digest too much food, there will be enough "energy" left to maintain and build health. It's important to understand the essential factors related to the quality of food and the amount of energy used for digestion. The best foods we can eat are the foods that supply the most nutrition but require the least amount of work for our bodies to digest and assimilate.

If we stop eating at nighttime, monitoring our hunger is so much easier. We can tell right away if we've eaten the right amount of food and the best quality food during the day. If we have, we probably won't be hungry. When we are always eating, it is harder to monitor this activity.

Emotional eating.

Without a doubt, our emotions can make us feel like we need to eat. Emotional eating is one of the biggest reasons we are such an obese nation. Turning to food for comfort has always been a device to escape our troubles.

If your hunger comes from reasons that are not related to nutrition, such as emotional dependence on food, they need be addressed accordingly. I meet too many people who do not address the real issue and never overcome their problems. There are emotional, mental, physical and spiritual causes. If your digestion and diet are fine but you feel hungry because of emotional issues they must be dealt with. Finding and treating the correct cause is often not addressed. People usually give far too much attention to the nutritional aspect but leave out the other areas to consider. It has been my experience that people suffer from all three areas but the most common of all is mentioned above: not getting the nutrients they are consuming. Many people seem to miss that issue, and that's why they are hungry all night.

Eating at nighttime is not the best thing to do for your health for many reasons. Why not deal with the problem before it becomes an issue and satisfy your body during the daytime when digestion is working at its best?

CHAPTER 12

LEARNING TO ADAPT

Change in the right direction.

One way or another, most of us have become used to some very unhealthful habits—junk food, staying up late, drinking too much coffee, whatever—and we actually enjoy them. That enjoyment came after years of consistent action and a lot of work. After all, most of us don't just change overnight.

Yet if we can get our bodies used to things that are bad for us, why can't we do it the other way? Why can't we get ourselves used to the good stuff, like healthful food, eating at the right times, and going to bed early? So if you are reading this and think you can't go without food late at night, or without eating six times a day, I'm here to tell you that you can!

People tell me it must be hard to eat a simple diet of healthful foods just a couple of times a day, and I always think how much harder it must be to have to think about food so much. When you spend time thinking about your next meal, what you're going to eat, where you're going to get it, and how to work your meals around your working hours so you'll get "enough" food—that's what seems like a lot of work to me. Trust me; been there, done that.

Pizza is the unofficial, official food of Brooklyn, N.Y., where I am from, and, when I was young, I lived on it. When I was a teenager, I worked for a financial brokerage firm on Wall Street. I spent my days among tons of people eating a lot of food. I felt like I had to be in the elite class of people eating the most pizza and drinking the most soda. Some days I would eat pizza for breakfast, lunch, dinner, and for a snack before bed.

As for soda, I was part of the Pepsi Generation, and to this day,

I am convinced they put a drug in Pepsi-Cola to make you want more after each sip. I could not eat pizza without a can of Pepsi, so that gives you an idea how much Pepsi I drank. I do not know how I was able to drink so much Pepsi and not "feel" sick, but just because I didn't feel sick didn't mean damage wasn't being done.

The first symptom of my Pepsi addiction revealed its ugly head at my annual trip to the dentist: 5 cavities. The following year: 10 cavities. The following year: 12 more cavities. That's 27 cavities in three years! And my dentist never said a word or tried to find out what might be causing all these cavities. I started to think he had stock in PepsiCo—although he had dishes full of candy sitting around the waiting room for his patients—or maybe I was drinking too much of the stuff? I began to wonder: If this soda was creating so much damage to my teeth, what was it doing to the rest of my body?

Up to that point in my life, I didn't dislike much, but the pain and the drill of the dentist were two things I didn't care for at all. To avoid the pain, I tried to convince myself I had a sugar addiction, but I weren't willing to give up the soda and the other sweets. I was just too addicted. If it wasn't for the dentist bills, I may have never been able to do it. Something had to be done, so as a first step, I decided to reduce the soda and replace it with fruit juice.

My switch to fruit drinks didn't eliminate the sugar, but it cut the amount down somewhat. I reduced the amount of soda I drank to one can a day, and then one can a week. But I never was able to get rid of the cravings, so I kept up the habit for a while. Finally, I was able to give up soda for six whole months. But then I was led to drink a soda. I took one sip and spit it out. It was terrible. I couldn't do it. I didn't even like the taste anymore. I never thought I'd find myself uttering these words, but it was too sweet. However, despite that, I did again become addicted to Pepsi, and it took me years to overcome my acquired habit.

My addiction to sugar was not natural; it was something

my body had adapted to over the years. No newborn baby is addicted to soda; replace mother's milk with cola, and the newborn baby will spit it out in an instant. Not only will our taste buds reject it, so will our body. But the more we persist, the more we persuade our taste buds to like it. Our body finally gives up and says, "OK, have it your way."

That is how the acquired habits of eating the wrong foods, eating too much food, and eating too often also take shape. If it's not the body or taste buds leading the way, it's the mind and emotions. I finally realized sugar wasn't my issue; eating too much sugar was my problem. So switching from Pepsi to Tang and Kool-Aid wasn't going to do the trick. Overcoming sugar addiction is hard enough, but I had a bigger issue to overcome: I was an overeater!

I have been teaching about health for many years now dealing with many sick people, and it is very seldom I run into someone who eats worse than I used to eat, or as much as I ate. On the average day, I would consume 7,000 calories, 300 grams of animal protein, and no produce because I hated fruits and vegetables. For a 150-pound man—for any man—that was a lot of food. My 33-inch waist didn't seem to be an issue, because my clothes fit well, but now I realize that, at 5'7", that was a real gut!

Now 20 years after overcoming my addiction to overeating, I'm 140 pounds with a 29-inch waist. Isn't it supposed to be the other way around? Aren't we supposed to put on weight as we age? No, we are not; I'm being facetious. I'm much happier with the results I'm getting than what passes as the norm in this country.

The human body has such an amazing ability to adapt to situations and just keep going. Most people are living under stress and may not even realize it, yet the body deals with it, adapts, and moves on, until it can't deal with the stress anymore. The problem is, just because we adapt and don't feel like we're under stress, doesn't mean damage isn't being done. I've met plenty of people who appear to be healthy. They eat as much as they want, whatever they want, whenever they want. Years later, though, they usually end up paying for it one way or another.

We acquire certain tastes or get used to living a certain way, and we become addicted to it, accept it as normal, and think that anyone who tries to get us to do things differently must be wrong.

I have worked with many people over the years, and I learned the hard way that there is a way out! There is a way to health.

The fact is that we can get ourselves so far from what should be, in almost every aspect of life: from money to debt, healthy to disease, happy to sad, and interested to bored. The good news is this proves we have the ability to change no matter what, so why not change in the right direction? Why not start now?

CHAPTER 13

THE POWER OF TEMPERANCE

The essence of the Daylight Diet

Temperance is the practice of moderation, although I have to say: I don't like to use the word "moderation" because, in my experience, people often define it incorrectly; one person's "moderate" is another person's "extreme." I think a better definition for temperance is restraint or self-control of excess, or maybe the opposite of excess. In other words, "moderation" may be doing less, compared to what you had been doing, but just because you're doing something less, doesn't mean you're practicing temperance.

These days, it seems many people are addicted to excess in so many facets of life. To those people, temperance not only sounds boring, but also limiting and unattainable. I understand this thinking, because I used to eat more than anyone I know. I haven't even met larger people who eat or ate more than I used to eat. My life was definitely one of excess eating. For me, life always had to be more. Temperance was the furthest thing from my mind.

Particularly regarding nutrition, I couldn't understand how less could be more. If something is good for you, don't you want to eat as much of it as you can? So I would eat and eat, not realizing the damage I was doing. The food was going to waste and taking my body down with it.

I do understand and respect the fact that, when it comes to chemistry and nutrition, there is no one, correct amount for everyone. We each come in different sizes and weights, and what is considered a little for one person can be a lot for another. However, based on our body type, age, current nutritional profile, climate, physical condition, and the quality of our food, there is a standard, moderate amount for each of us, and it shouldn't be based on how we feel or what we believe, but purely on the fact that our body needs a certain amount of nutrients to survive. Any amount above that is going to impact our health, and not in a good way. Many of us would be surprised to find out we are eating far more than we need to be; others simply wouldn't care.

Less is more.

We also have to be careful not to decide how much we need based on our weight; muscle weighs more than fat, so forget about that excuse or loophole. Also, excess, stored fat in the gut is never good for us. If you are carrying around extra fat, it means you are taking in more than you need. There is a difference between the body being able to use fat for energy and being overweight. You do not have to carry a spare tire around your waist for your body to produce the energy it needs to thrive.

In his book *The Natural Food for Man*, Dr. Hereward Carrington talks about the correct amount of food for us: "Every individual should restrict himself to the smallest quantity that he finds, from careful investigation and experiment, will meet the wants of his system, knowing that whatever is more than this is harmful."

Luigi Cornaro was a man who lived 102 years, and his secret for a long life was very simple: "Man should live up to the simplicity dictated by nature, which teaches us to be content with little, and accustom ourselves to eat no more than is absolutely necessary to support life, remembering that all excess causes disease and leads to death."

Until Cornaro was 35, he ate just as much as everyone else—until he got very sick. His doctors even told him to prepare to die. Cornaro began eating less, and he did die—67 years later, at the age of 102. And this was in 1566!

Cornaro came to the same conclusion many other centenarians come to:

If temperance can heal the sick, then it must also have the power to preserve our health and strength.

All the major popular spiritual leaders in history taught temperance, especially when it comes to diet. In my book *Health According to the Scriptures*, I talk about how Yeshua (Jesus) warned His disciples that, just prior to His second coming, the state of the world would be as it was just prior to The Flood: Eating and drinking would be carried to excess, and the world would be given up to pleasure.

In her Christian health writings, Ellen G. White wrote: "The world is largely given up to the indulgence of appetite; and the disposition to follow worldly customs will bring us into bondage to perverted habits—habits that will make us more and more like the doomed inhabitants of Sodom. I see reason enough for the present state of degeneracy and mortality in the world. Blind passion controls reason, and every high consideration is, what many sacrificed to lust."

In my books and lectures, I often talk about the types of foods that are best for the body: raw, ripe, fresh, organic, living foods! However, when and how often we eat has just as much of an impact on our health, maybe even more. I know many people who eat a lousy diet but don't overeat, and they seem to be doing somewhat OK. And I know a lot of people who overeat healthful foods, but aren't doing so well.

Health doesn't begin with what we add to our diet, but with what we leave out. If overeating is causing us so many issues, doesn't it seem sensible and wise to stop overeating?

Live long and prosper.

Many studies have shown the superiority of a low-calorie diet. Eating less sounds pretty simple, but it is a challenge to accomplish because we live in a world of excess. The fact is, the body becomes more efficient and develops better health if less food is eaten. Just take a look around the world, and find the oldest people in the world. They are usually of the poorer classes and can't afford to indulge in excess. Regardless of what they eat, they all seem to share the same secret to great health: they are light eaters.

I have read great stories of people in the past who lived lives far exceeding the average, and in just about every case, their great age was attributed to eating very little. But are those stories true? Maybe or maybe not. Tales from the past about people's great age are often fabricated; however, more and more people are living beyond 100 years, and the ones who claim they eat very little seem to be thriving and look and act so much younger. Sometimes, it's just hard to believe they're that old unless you've seen them with your own eyes. Maybe those stories from the past have some validity.

I personally know a great example of what we can accomplish when we eat less. He is my friend Bernando LaPallo. I met Bernando when he was 104. He was in great health and very active. He appeared to be in his 60s, if I had to take a guess. When I found out he was 104, I had to find out more about his fountain of youth. Now, four years later, at 108, Bernando and I have become friends, and he has come out with a book letting everyone know his keys to great health. In his book *Age Less, Live More*, he shares his three golden rules for great health and long life:

- Maintain a positive, optimistic outlook on life.
- Be active, move, and exercise.
- Eat natural foods in the right amounts; do not overeat.

There are so few examples of people achieving great health at any great age, not because it's not possible, but because people are not aware or not willing to live according to those three rules. We are brought up to eat in excess. Our society and culture make it more challenging to resist food. We each have to understand and believe temperance is key, and we need to be temperate in all things, especially eating.

Of all the health writers I've studied, each preached a message of temperance in diet. Here is what Hilton Hotema says in his book, *Man's Higher Consciousness*:

"Life is Creation's greatest treasure for Man in the flesh, and most men should enjoy it much longer than they do. This can easily be done by learning the body's simple requirements and living in harmony with that knowledge.

"All living creatures are ruled by the same laws of Creation, but they do not all live in harmony with those laws. Those that come the closest to it are those that live the longest in proportion to the length of time required for them to reach maturity of physical development.

"There are many reasons, most of them preventable, why people die young and why hospitals are filled with the sick, while others are seldom ill and live three to ten times longer. It would logically seem that living creatures with the higher intelligence should be the ones to live the nearest to the requirements of the laws of Creation; but in action it seems to work the other way: The more intelligent creatures being those who appear to stray the farthest from the straight and narrow path which leads unto life (Matthew 7:13-14)."

Here is what Ellen White has to say about intemperate eating in her book Diet and Foods:

"Intemperance in eating, even of healthful food, will have an injurious effect upon the system, and will blunt the mental and moral faculties. Nearly all the members of the human family eat more than their system requires. This excess decays and becomes a putrid mass. If more food, even of a simple quality, is placed in the stomach than the living machinery requires, this surplus becomes a burden. The system makes desperate efforts to dispose of it, and this extra work causes a tired, weary feeling. Some who are continually eating call this all-gone feeling hunger, but it is caused by the overworked condition of the digestion organs."

The majority of us eat much more than we need to. The result is a lower quality of life. By simply following the plan laid out for you in the Daylight Diet, by eating the right foods temperately, you too can live a long, healthful life.

But temperance—eating fewer calories—is the essence of the Daylight Diet. Eating less takes very little thought. Simply eat only two small-to-medium meals a day at the correct times. Don't snack in between meals. Stop eating at nighttime. A very simple idea.

CHAPTER 14

ENDURANCE AND ENTHUSIASM

It's all in the planning.

In high school, I was on the track team and was a long-distance runner. Our coach always told us that the most important rule to remember in long-distance running was to "pace yourself." If I started off too quickly, I would run out of steam before the end of the race. Endurance is the key to success, not only in long-distance racing, but also in all aspects of health. When you adapt the Daylight Diet, it's important to remember to pace yourself, or rather, pace your meals.

It is helpful to always remember that, if you consume enough nutrients in the daytime, you won't be hungry at night. The more wisely you stock up nutrients during the daytime, the more comfortable you will be mentally and physically during the nighttime. It all comes down to eating in a way so that your body will be digesting and distributing nutrients evenly throughout the day and night.

Once you determine how many meals to eat in a day, you then have to decide when it's best to eat them. For example, if you decide to eat just one meal a day, having that meal first thing in the morning is probably not a wise thing to do; it will be so much more difficult to pace yourself if you have to go the whole day and night with no food. It would make more sense to have that meal during the middle of the day.

If you decide to eat two meals a day, you'd want to space them out—preferably at the third and ninth hour after sunrise, as we discussed earlier — and not eat them back to back. Whether you decide to eat three meals or even one meal a day, thinking and planning ahead is going to help you be successful; otherwise, you may run out of steam and quit. Give yourself the best chance to be successful.

Some people who do not understand this may worry about where they will get enough energy if they do not eat at nighttime. They need to understand that, when you get sufficient rest and sleep at night, your body recharges so you will have enough energy and endurance throughout the next day. This is why not overeating is so vital to health: When you eat more than you need, or at the wrong times, it affects your sleep and your body's entire schedule the next day. In other words, being healthy and sticking to a schedule comes down to the quality of your sleep. The Daylight Diet puts the body in a position to get the best rest each night and to stay on a schedule that will consistently help you thrive!

Another way to understand this is to think about plugging in your cell phone each night before you go to bed so it can recharge. In the morning, if it's had enough time to recharge, it works fine. But if you don't plug it in one night, or, if you get to bed late and don't plug it in until late, it won't have a fully charged battery, and it will be just a matter of time before it will automatically shut off. When we get sufficient sleep, we are recharging our battery. We want it to be fully charged when we wake up so we don't automatically shut down during the day.

We conserve our energy and produce healing from sleep. As we discussed before, food is a stimulant that gives us a quick burst of what feels like energy but in reality is stimulation. If we don't get enough sleep night after night, we're not just losing energy; we're also throwing off our schedule the next day. Health is all about conserving energy, and that's exactly what the Daylight Diet does for you.

Planning ahead puts your mind and body in the best situation to get the well-needed rest and the proper amount of nourishment at the right times: What food is on hand? What appointments do you have that day? What people will you be with? Where and when will you shop? Planning your schedule and sticking to it is going to help you achieve your goal more than anything else you do.

The importance of passion

I find that people who adapt the Daylight Diet and learn to plan their schedules and stick to them, have passion and joy in their lives. They understand what they have to do, and they do it. A big difference between those who succeed at the Daylight Diet and those who fail is enthusiasm. It seems to make all the difference in the world. If you're not enthusiastic about what you are doing, you're not going to enjoy it, but also you're not going to fully understand the benefits you can reap from it.

I wasn't the fastest long-distance runner on my high school track team. I wasn't in the best shape compared to my other teammates. But my enthusiasm to cross that finish line ahead of them motivated me never to give up during those times when it seemed like there was no hope that I could even finish the race. My enthusiasm made me successful.

Are you excited to become a Daylight Dieter? The measure of your enthusiasm will foretell your level of success.

Look to the future.

And if you fail? Do not let failure stop you; instead, let it motivate you. I've been eating a Daylight Diet for a while now, and people often ask me if I am 100 percent compliant and successful at it. Right now, I can pretty much say, yes: except for rare occasions, I do not eat after a certain time and never when it's dark outside. However, if I slip up, I don't let that upset me.

Some people will throw away all of their hard work—days, weeks, and even months of success—because they mess up once or twice. You have to look at the big picture. If you treat your body great most of the time, you will thrive. I'm not giving you an excuse not to stay on the Daylight Diet; I'm just putting things in perspective. After all, most people abuse their bodies every day, and they survive. You have to put things in perspective. Life is not about being 100 percent perfect; it's about enjoying what you're doing and doing what works best for you.

What you did in the past does not matter—you no longer have control over that. What's important now is how you intend to take care of yourself in the future.

When I awake each morning after a good night's sleep, I feel amazingly energized and extra excited about the day ahead. I plan my day so I understand what has to be done. It makes it much easier to be enthusiastic about everything I have to do. Enjoying life comes down to how we approach it.

Have a plan, make a schedule, pace yourself, and you will thrive.

CHAPTER 15

THE FORMULA FOR HEALTH

Good digestion equals good health

In my last book, *The Raw Food Formula for Health*, I explained how the body creates health by conserving energy. Good digestion helps the body conserve the most energy, so anything you can do to keep digestion strong will keep you healthy and strong, too.

The key to this formula is to avoid adding any unnecessary digestive work to the cleansing and healing the body already has to do every day. With the Daylight Diet, we add one more piece to the puzzle that is good health. The Daylight Diet will fuel ideal digestion and help you achieve the formula for health.

Being successful at the Daylight Diet will be much easier if you understand you do not need much food to thrive. The nutrients in food will nourish the body, but it takes the body a lot of work to digest the food and extract those nutrients from the food. The body works even harder to get rid of the parts of the food it cannot use; this is known as waste. Getting a good night's rest and taking a break every night from eating help the body conserve its energy so that it can fight disease. If the body does not have enough energy, or if there is obstruction (waste), illness can then take hold.

The Formula

The formula for health, invented by Arnold Ehret, is not difficult to understand:

Power - Obstruction = Vitality, or V = P - O

"Power" is health, or as I prefer to refer to it, "energy." I don't mean energy as in stimulation, but rather the energy you get when you've had the proper sleep and nutrition. "Obstruction" is disease. And "vitality" is wellness, or the level of health we experience, so:

Health - Disease=Wellness, or W = H - D

In other words, your degree of wellness or vitality is what's left of your health when you "subtract" any sickness or discomfort. For example, if you're a very healthy person and you happen to get a cold, you still have a good supply of overall wellness. But if you don't eat right, and you're not sleeping enough, and then you get a cold, you'll have less vitality and ability to heal. Obviously, the healthier you are, the more vitality you will have to help you when you get sick.

As long as the body is able to maintain enough power/health to remove the obstruction/disease, there is going to be some degree of vitality/wellness. If the obstruction/disease becomes greater than your power/health, you won't have the energy to get rid of the obstruction. The greater the obstruction, the more likely the disease will reach an advanced stage.

So the state of our health is determined by the degree of this vital energy we have left after the body has used its power to get rid of the waste. If the body runs out of energy to supply the power, waste will build up more quickly. Because the body no longer has enough energy to eliminate the buildup of toxic substances, an excess amount of toxins accumulates in the blood; soon, you're experiencing the first stage of disease.

If Power - Obstruction = Vitality, or the amount of health we have is equal to Power - Obstruction, too little power and too much obstruction will put us in a very diseased state. This is the essence of the Formula for Health, and, as we'll see, it can help you understand how a high-quality raw food diet, sufficient sleep, and detoxification can keep the obstructions in check and your vitality soaring.

The source of power

Power comes from all the gifts our Creator has given us that so many of us take for granted. These gifts make our body a wonderfully strong and amazing machine. The air we breathe; the water we drink; fresh, high-quality food; and sunlight are just some of the many gifts we receive every day. Proper use of these gifts can make you stronger, increasing your power without using your innate energy to do it.

Many daily pressures we experience—poor diet, environmental and emotional stress, or even spiritual confusion and doubt—consume energy/vitality, zap the body's power production. Unfortunately, there's no true test to conclude how much energy we have or don't have. Science can determine how much vitality we have only to a degree, based on our organ functions and stress levels, but since there are many other factors that indicate vitality, or lack if it, science cannot provide reliable measurements. The good news is, the body stores energy, and very few people will ever reach energy deprivation as long as they follow nature's laws.

One way to maintain your energy is to heal the body simply, by allowing it to do so, because, once we interfere, the body is forced to expend energy to deal with the interference. As you will begin to understand, the key to conserving energy is to rid yourself of obstructions through long periods without food, such as on the Daylight Diet.

A common misconception is that energy or vitality means stimulation. But stimulation is not vitality. Rather, it is a false source of energy with levels that go up and down depending on what we eat or don't eat. Real energy is always there until we do something to use it up. Health, or energy, is not achieved by what we add, but by what we get rid of. Health is not about eating more highly stimulating foods, but eating fewer of them.

High-quality nutrition, along with a clean internal environment, will help create and conserve energy/vitality. The key to health from a physical standpoint is to take in the required nutrients while using as little power as possible to digest it, and then keep the body's internal environment as clean as possible. Raw fruits and vegetables do just that.

A consistent flow of energy in our body will keep us healthy, vibrant, and excited about life. The more energy we have, the more power we can produce. The first sign of energy drain is the first sign of disease. Take, for example, a sports car: No matter how powerful the engine in the car, without gasoline, the car will not go anywhere.

Fruits and vegetables require the least amount of the body's energy to digest, yet they provide the most nutrients. In other words, you get more bang for your buck with fruits and vegetables than any other foods. They are your best source of energy, as long as, of course, you don't overeat or eat at nighttime. Overeating—and eating at the wrong times—zaps energy.

Overeating and obstruction

If we know that obstruction causes a depletion of body energy, what can we do to prevent it? The most common cause of obstruction is eating too much food (especially at the wrong times). This makes overeating, in my opinion, the leading cause of disease. The only thing that comes close to causing as much disease, in my opinion, is lack of sleep or insufficient sleep (often a result of overeating and eating at nighttime).

Overeating creates obstruction—too much food in the system cuts into our power base because our body has to use energy to store or expel the excess—and lack of sleep, or "undersleeping," as I like to call it, does not give the body enough time to recharge, causing a lack of power. Not enough power and too much obstruction put us into a state of disease.

Another major issue with overeating is that it leads to the first stage of disease: constipation. When we eat too much food, or we eat the wrong foods at the incorrect times, we are no longer assisting the body in doing its job; in fact, we're working against it. Here is what Ehret had to say about it in his book *Mucusless Diet Healing System*:

> "(Constipation is) a clogging up of the entire pipe system of the human body. Any special system is therefore merely an extraordinary local constipation by more accumulated mucus at this particular place. Special accumulation points are the tongue, the stomach and particularly the entire digestive tract. This last is the real and deeper cause of bowel constipation. The average person has as much as ten pounds of uneliminated feces in the bowels continually, poisoning the blood stream and the entire system. Think of it!
>
> "Every sick person has a more or less mucus-clogged system, such mucus being derived from undigested and uneliminated, unnatural food substances accumulated from childhood on. The average man has not the slightest idea what the necessary eliminative process is, what time it requires, how and how often his diet must be changed, what it means to cleanse the body of the terrible quantities of waste he has accumulated in his body during his life."

Disease is simply an effort by the body to eliminate waste created by overeating and eating at the wrong times. By following the principles of the Daylight Diet, you will always be one step ahead of disease.

CHAPTER 16

THE DAILY DETOX

A clean body needs less food.

Eating for pleasure has replaced the concept of eating for nourishment, and this has led to a society that consumes more food more often than necessary. The most outward sign of this is an epidemic of overweight people; an even more common one is lack of energy.

Overeating adds waste, or mucus, to our system. Waste creates toxic gas—a result of the waste trapped in our intestines—which is released into our bloodstream, leading to many deadly problems. Once there is a buildup of mucus, the body can no longer perform the way it was meant to or thrive on very little amounts of food. The first step in preparing the body for less food is to stop the buildup of the mucus and let the body do its job to get rid of it. The Daylight Diet is the divine way to eat to help our body clean out each night after we stop eating to avoid the buildup of waste.

The cause of illness

In his book *The Cause and Cure of Human Illness,* Arnold Ehret writes:

> "My first major point is that every illness, without exception, is an attempt by the body to eliminate mucus and, in advanced stages, pus (disintegrated blood). Every healthy organism of course must contain a certain amount of naturally occurring mucus, called lymph, the fatty mucus-like substance of the colon. Every medical expert dealing with cathartic problems, from a harmless runny nose to pneumonia and tuberculosis, will attest to this fact.

"But we are examining here a very unnatural and unhealthy mucus condition which is epidemic in modern society. The body's attempt to eliminate excess mucus is not always obvious in disease of the ears, eyes, skin diseases, stomach problems, heart trouble, rheumatism, arthritis, etc., not to mention in mental disturbances. And yet excess mucus is the main cause of the problem. Mucus, which can no longer be eliminated through natural means, enters the blood and reappears at a location where the blood circulation is reduced (perhaps because of a strong chill) as heat symptom, an inflammation, a pain, or maybe a fever produced by the body.

"I am not saying that mucus is always and exclusively the cause of all diseases, but I do maintain that mucus is the common basic factor of all diseases. There can be many other causes of disease and I do not deny them, but mucus will be involved in each and every case."

Cleanse and detox

That's what's so wonderful about the Daylight Diet. You eat less, so there's less waste, and every night your body automatically goes into a cleanse mode and detoxifies in a healthful way. That's every single night!

Your body always defaults to cleaning and rebuilding when you're not eating and the body has already digested what you have eaten. When you overeat and eat too many meals in a day, the body is always digesting and has less time to go through a cleansing and rebuilding cycle. Then your health declines. The longer you can go each night with no food or water, the more healing and cleansing can take place.

We should do our best to assist the body's natural process of *detoxification*. Through herbal formulas, colonics, enemas, fasting, and other methods, we rid the body of excess waste. Once the body starts to eliminate long-stored waste from the body, detoxification begins. In my opinion, the more often we help the body cleanse itself, the better chance we have of preventing the common diseases that so many suffer from today. Whenever you reflect on health, remember that, although nutrition is important, it's the cleansing that makes the difference.

But also keep in mind each of us is unique; what may be good for one person may not be good for another. For example, when I first began eating a raw foods diet, my body was very toxic and had a lot of waste to get rid of. (My waist was 33 inches, and I'm only 5'7". That's not good!) Back then, there was no way I could have gone 15 hours a night without food, because I was in the habit of eating often; after just a few hours without food, I would start to feel bad. I had to cleanse slowly and build up my body. Years later, I'm now at the point where I can get through the night and go many more hours without food and not miss it. Years ago, going without food for a short time would not have been comfortable for me, but today, it is a pleasure. I'm not boasting. I'm not special. Everyone can get to this point, and the quickest and smartest way to do it is to adopt the Daylight Diet.

Dr. Fred Bisci is living proof that, once we are healthy, we do not need much food to thrive. Dr. Bisci told me about an experiment he did for eight years to see how little he could eat and still be healthy. (When Fred was a young man, he was an Olympic class weightlifter. He weighed more than 230 pounds and ate often.) He eventually adopted a raw vegan diet, and, after many years of eating little, he conducted this experiment. Fred gradually reduced his intake of food over time and got to a point where he needed only a very small amount of food each day. He ate a low-calorie, nutrient-dense but nourishing diet to see how long he could exist on this type of a lifestyle. Fred was surprised it took so many years to come up with his answer, but he reached the point were he got his result. In his book *Your Healthy Journey*, Dr. Bisci writes:

"I learned that systematic under-eating is the surest way of improving your health, giving both immediate and long-term results.

When your body adjusts to systematic under-eating, it slows down your metabolic rate, which slows down the aging process, but at the same time you get all the nutrients you need."

Dr. Bisci is very secretive about his process because he understands that reducing food intake is so individualized. One person may be able to reduce his calories very quickly and gain health; another may have to take months or years to do so. If a person tries to reduce the amount of food too quickly before his body can adjust on a chemical level, it can do more harm than good. He warns people that on a high quality diet of raw, ripe, fresh, organic foods, the body becomes an amazingly efficient biological machine; however, you can't rush the process. If you force yourself to systematically undereat, and don't allow your body to adapt on a chemical level, you'll become undernourished.

Even following the Daylight Diet, which I think is the safest plan to reduce food intake, it may take years for your body to adapt completely to the final stage of the plan, but everyone can and should start with the Stage 1 as soon as possible. The more toxic the body, the longer it takes to get to the ultimate stage; just as the body took years to adapt to eating so much, it will take the body years to adapt to less food. The healthier you are, the less time it will take. But be assured that, over time, your body chemistry will change, and you will gradually require less food, less often.

When you go on the Daylight Diet, move at your own pace. There's no need to jump to the later stages in a short time; it can be too challenging and maybe too hard on the body. However, if you take your time and consistently take steps in the right direction, you can achieve the same results in a more comfortable manner.

How do I know my pace?

Like anything else, you want to advance quickly enough to see results, but slowly enough so you enjoy the changes. You know you've hit your pace when you are eating less food and find you are enjoying the feeling. There still may be minor discomfort during the process, but as long as you have the knowledge about how the body cleanses, you will enjoy the results. If the discomfort becomes too uncomfortable, just go back to eating a little more until your body is ready for less. Unless you are in serious stages of disease, there is no reason to rush the process. Just keep moving in the right direction, and you will be fine.

It is not always easy to figure out what direction you are moving in because detoxifying and deficiency can have the same symptoms. To figure out which is happening to you, it helps to keep a log monitoring your bowel and sleep habits and your blood chemistry. We'll discuss this in the next part of this book.

So how much food do we really need?

It's very sad that Americans are so conditioned to overconsume food, but it is no longer an issue only in America. All over the world, people are eating more than ever before. Generation X has become Generation XL, and the baby boomers continued the trend. I love the way Dr. Lewis writes about how we treat our bodies. It was written in 1870, so some of the foods may seem odd, but regardless, we continue to treat ourselves the same way today:

"I have often wondered what the stomach must say to itself while an ordinary meal is coming down. This stomach knows perfectly well what it needs. It asks at breakfast a moderate piece of steak, a slice or two of stale bread, and a baked potato. Now, just stand by and see what comes down. First, a great mass of greasy buckwheat cakes, now, a swash of scalding hot coffee, again buckwheats, more coffee, sausage, hot biscuit saturated with melted butter, buckwheats, coffee, sausage, hot biscuit, and so on and so on for half an hour. And here we have an enormous mass of hot, greasy, doughy, indigestible stuffs swimming in hot coffee.

"The stomach asks at dinner, roast beef or mutton, with bread, potatoes and other vegetables. Now, what is the conglomeration that comes rushing down that red canal? Turtle soup, fish, beef, duck, plum pudding, pie, nuts, raisins, coffee, and several condiments; with this hotchpotch, ice water, ice cream and wine. For supper, the stomach asks for nothing, and it gets hot biscuit, butter, cake, preserves, and strong tea.

"Boardinghouses are beginning to occupy a large place in our city and town life. Delicate women, with scrofula, congregate in these places, gorge themselves after the above fashion, and for exercise wear a tight corset and sit over the register. I cannot think of but one good result that comes of this, and that is a large class of very respectable citizens. The doctors get a good living out of it."

I believe that, once our body is healthy and cleansed, we need very little food, as long as it is good quality. I think most people could reduce their food intake by half and be healthier. Eating two meals and following the Daylight Diet is the most healthful and natural way to do this. It is the way we have been designed to eat.

"But where will I get my calories?" I hear this so often from people who attend my lectures and read my books. Calorie counting is not something you need to concern yourself with, because one calorie is not the same as another. For example, 500 calories from candy doesn't give you the same nutrient package as 500 calories from spinach. If you are only concerned about calories, you will end up with other health problems. What's important is the type of food, when it's consumed, and how easily the body can process and utilize it. Science confirms that a reduced-calorie diet is more healthful and helps you live longer, but those scientists weren't talking about calories from just any place. If you are concerned with counting calories, you have to make your calories count.

It's not the amount of food or number of calories that's important; it's how much of what you eat the body actually uses. The more nutritious food, the less of it you need to eat. The cleaner your body, the more efficiently it will extract nutrients from the food. Excess will cause trouble. The more efficient the body is working, the quicker it will get rid of waste, and the healthier you will be. The longer you eat raw, ripe, fresh, organic food, the greater your ability to thrive on a lot less food.

If we keep our bodies clean on a cellular level, the more efficiently it can do its job, and it needs only a very little amount of food to thrive.

The reason we require less food when we are clean is because a clean colon improves the absorption of nutrients, increases peristaltic action of the intestines (keeping waste moving through), and conserves the body's energy. I've met people all over the world who have experienced rapid healing and relief from a clean colon.

In addition to colon cleansing, cleaning your body internally, at the cellular level, requires not only detoxifying but also fasting. Fasting–a diet of water or fresh juice–is particularly cleansing because it helps the body release toxic gases that otherwise would find their way into cells. There are numerous ways to expel toxins. I think the best way is the Daylight Diet.

CHAPTER 17

EMOTIONS, ENVIRONMENT, AND SOCIAL CHANGES

Dealing with your friends, your family, and yourself

We are in a society where we need to be stimulated by an alarm clock to wake up, need a caffeinated drink to stay awake, and need mental stimulation such as TV to stay interested—or shall I say programmed—in life. We use tons of make-up and perfume to make ourselves fashionable and smell good, and we have plastic surgery to have a "healthy" appearance. People are finally learning that these things don't improve our self-esteem; neither are they healthful.

Today, people are much more interested in taking responsibility for their health than ever before. The rising cost of health care and obesity from high-fat junk foods are motivating people to pay more attention to preventing disease instead of dealing with it after the fact. People are finally waking up, and they want to be healthy.

We still have a long way to go, of course, but at least I am no longer looked upon as crazy when I tell people I don't use a microwave oven or drink coffee. Vegetarian diets are now accepted, and the living foods diet, also known as the raw foods diet, is quickly becoming the new, healthful way to eat.

Even the chemical food companies are realizing that a shift is taking place. The companies are changing their advertising and marketing—or shall I say programming— adding words such as "fat-free," "natural," "healthy," and "made with real fruits and vegetables" to their labels. Don't be fooled: Many of these products are the same products with new advertising.

There was a time when people were very active and ate healthfully. It was only a few hundred years ago that everyone's diet was mostly fruits and vegetables that weren't sprayed with toxic chemicals. One of the most valued jobs was "farmer." Today, that job may have lost value in people's eyes, but it is still among the most important. Big business has tried to take away that value, by hybridizing and modifying seeds and actually making it much harder for the small farmer to stay in business.

I hear many people preface statements today with *"when I get sick,"* rather than *"if I get sick."* They don't even realize what they are saying. It wasn't much different for me, though. As long as there was a doctor, and I had insurance, it didn't matter what I put into my body.

Once people get sick, their thoughts on the matter change. They don't want to deal with the pain. It kind of reminds me of drinking. People go out with friends and innocently have a few drinks and a lot of fun. But a few drinks become more and more, and before they know it, they wake with a hangover and promise to never drink again. But sure enough, a few days pass, and they're drinking again.

Do you know what the definition of "insanity" is? It's doing the same thing over and over and expecting different results. If you want to change the results, you have to change the action.

If we want to be healthy, we must change what we put in our bodies. If you have a sugar- or fat-related illness and go on a vegetarian, vegan, or raw diet but continue to overeat fatty and sugary foods, you are going to continue to suffer from illness.

Nothing takes away our youthfulness and energy more quickly than carrying around too much weight. Being overweight, once considered odd, has become the norm in our country, even for children. If we want to get control over weight gain, the Daylight Diet is the answer.

We discussed earlier why we feel we have to eat at nighttime—because we are used to low-quality food, and our bodies aren't getting the right nutrients. And we have touched on emotional eating because some of us use food to comfort ourselves. But there is more to emotional eating than comfort, and if people can get these next two root issues under control, the Daylight Diet should be a breeze.

There are two main areas of our lives that we must feel good about if we don't want to overeat and/or eat late at night: our money and our health. Poor health and the lack of money are two of the biggest contributors to depression, and when we get depressed, we eat—especially at night. We can't get these things off our minds, and then we have trouble getting a good night's sleep. So, instead of doing something productive about our problems, we run to food for comfort.

If you want an easier time achieving the Daylight Diet, put a plan together to improve your health and become debt free. Some advantages of the Daylight Diet, of course, are that you will gain health, plus you'll spend less money on food. So it can help you overcome these issues, which further motivates you to stay on the Daylight Diet.

When your emotions are under control, you make better decisions and feel better about everything.

Your money or your life

Money, or, rather, the lack of it, can destroy us emotionally. People in debt are usually very depressed. There are some very valid reasons why we sometimes spend more money than we make—emergencies, medical bills, etc.—however, most people just do not have control of their spending. Credit cards are a debt trap, too.

You may question why I have included a discussion about money in a book about diet, but I can tell you from experience that a person who does not take good care of their financial life is usually not disciplined enough to eat a Daylight Diet.

This doesn't mean someone in this position cannot overcome the issue. I've been in debt, and I know that you don't have to be debt free to be emotionally happy. What you must do, though, is be working on the debt and have a plan and a budget so that you feel in control. It's such a great feeling, knowing you don't owe anyone anything! Then you will have an easy time with all your goals, including the Daylight Diet.

(I also highly recommend listening to Dave Ramsey, author and radio and TV host, who has helped hundreds of people get out of debt. Check out his schedule and his books at www.daveramsey.com)

Exercise is wise

An exercise or fitness program also will make you feel better and can help lift depression. I struggled with nighttime eating my whole life until I realized how much better I felt, and how much less I ate, when I was involved in a regular fitness program.

That's right; I said how much less I ate while on a fitness program. Most people associate exercise with eating more so they can "keep their fuel up." We all need some fitness in our life, but it's not wise to exercise more just so you can eat more. To a degree, that's just another form of eating disorder. We've already discussed adrenaline rush, so people who are involved in extreme sports that require tremendous amounts of fuel or energy might want to reconsider what it's really doing to the body. If you are training to run a once-in-a-lifetime marathon race, that's one thing, but making a living out of extreme events really is not conducive to a long, healthy life.

You should get used to a regular fitness program; however, you don't have to do anything special or expensive: you just have to move. Walking, jogging, rebounding—whatever you enjoy. Do not do something you don't enjoy because it will be just a matter of time before you fail. There are so many forms of exercise you should have no problem finding out what types you love the best. If you start to get bored, you can always find something else. Mixing it up keeps it interesting and fun.

While we are on the topic of exercise, I also think we should exercise only when it is daylight. At nighttime, our bodies are winding down to resting mode. Exercising when it's dark outside will create as much harm to the body as eating when it is dark outside. I used to be in the gym working out at 5 a.m. every morning. What a mistake I was making!

Once you are in a good position emotionally, you will be able to achieve all your goals. Of course, there are other personal things that emotionally drive us to overeat and eat late at night. If we are in the world, our emotional health is at risk all the time. We must have control over our emotions to be safe. Losing control of emotions leads to addictions, which can become very harmful.

Environmental protection

Our environment is made up of everything from the people we spend our time with to the places we live and work. The human body is different from most other living things because it has an amazing ability to adapt to various environments. This can be good or bad, depending on the environment. A salt-water fish cannot survive in fresh water, and a tropical fruit cannot grow in the cold. These things are very sensitive to their environments, but we are not. We have to remember that just because we have the ability to adapt, doesn't mean that's what is best for us. If we are adapting to an unhealthful environment, we may not feel the effects right away, but eventually we will become a victim to the negative thing in our environment, even though we didn't realize what was taking place.

The health of your body can never be any better than the health of your environment. I was born and raised in New York City. It was loud, crowded, dirty, and fast. As I got older and wiser and searched for a more healthful place to live, I looked all over the world. I traveled often, making up quickly for the travel I didn't get as a child. The first time I left my home, it seemed weird to be in a new place, but the more often I left, the more comfortable I felt in the new environment, especially if I had visited more than once. A brand new environment can seem quite shocking, to say the least.

It works the same way with health and the body. Drastic changes in diet or lifestyle can shock the body, but if the adjustment is made slowly and often, the body has an easier time adapting.

We have adapted to eating an amount of food never meant for our bodies to handle. At the expense of our growing stomachs and inflamed organs, we keep pushing the envelope to see how far we can take it. When we eat, we should finish our meal before we are full so we can get up and comfortably walk away from the table. Instead, we overindulge knowingly and, being aware we ate too much, say, "I can't eat another bite." But then dessert comes to the table, and we eat many more bites. Now instead of freely and comfortably leaving the table, we find ourselves holding our stomachs and leaving the room in pain, feeling tired and drowsy.

The human body can adapt to eating this way and will have to work hard to overcome this adaptation, because it is no longer about nutrition or nourishment but a matter of health versus disease, or life verses death. Gluttony leads to health issues that will haunt us forever if we don't put the fork down and step away from the table before we eat so much that we are falling asleep, another common trend that is happening today. Seriously, we have to stop eating so much, or we will surely regret it later in life.

There is no reason why we shouldn't be able to eat two meals a day and be perfectly healthy, but we have adapted to eating three or more times a day, so now we are sick. We have become used to spending our time and money thinking about food, looking for food, preparing our food, and recovering from the damage we created from our food. We can no longer enjoy our life. The temporary pleasure our taste buds enjoy has replaced the joy that should fill the rest of our lives.

Others' reactions

The longer I eat only two meals a day and see the benefits, the more I question how I was ever able to eat any more. After not eating at nighttime for a while, I couldn't imagine eating late in the day, let alone when it is dark outside. Why was I able to realize this, but other people cannot?

The reactions I got from people when I told them about my plans for the Daylight Diet were no surprise. My family already thought I was nuts because I ate a raw food, vegan diet. They are right in one respect: you are what you eat, and I did consume nuts! So dealing with their reactions wasn't too difficult, other than my dad thinking I was going to starve to death, or others, who weren't sure they could hang out with me anymore because the only time we seem to be able to do anything is when it involves going out to eat dinner.

The reactions from my friends weren't too bad. Most of them knew I was healthy, and it didn't surprise them that I found a new experiment to improve the quality of my health. They were supportive but more interested to learn more, just as the general health community seemed to be. I started a blog, giving updates to keep everyone informed. To everyone's surprise, I didn't lose much weight, but I looked better than I ever had. My wife noticed the positive changes right away. I'll never forget when she told me the whites of my eyes were as clear as ivory. I had more energy eating this way than I've ever had before. All it took was to stop eating late at night.

Of all the reactions I got, the biggest surprise and the most joyful one was from my wife. I thought she was going to have a fit when I announced to her I wasn't going to eat at nighttime. "No more going out to eat for dinner?" was what I thought I was going to hear. But to my pleasant surprise, she was all for it.

She jokingly said, "You already eat a boring diet, so fine." I'm sure the books on my nightstand had something to do with her willingness to give up the late night, candlelight dinners. She must have peeked at a few of those books, because in a short time she was willing to give it a try herself.

As for dealing with the general public, eating an unpopular way has never been an issue to me. If I couldn't find something to eat, I just wouldn't. Not a big deal.

I know many people have different lifestyles, and I've heard all the excuses. Let me give you my answer to these responses, and then how you handle them is up to you.

My brother-in-law is such a nice man, and a man of much willpower. I was excited to learn just before he married my sister that he'd given up smoking. I prayed this would rub off on my sister. (That hasn't happened yet, but it's still a strong prayer.)

As strong willed as my brother-in-law is, when it comes to diet and health, he is the Anti-Paul. He eats nothing green and eats most of his calories late at night. I once asked him to make a few diet changes, nothing too radical, just maybe add some fruit smoothies, hoping to one day get him to try to add greens to the smoothies. He had lots of excuses why it would be impossible for him to do that.

I love him and my sister dearly, and it hurts to see how they're harming themselves, but there does come a time when you have to step back and just pray. They know what I do and how I can help them, and when they are ready, I will be there for them, but until then, I will continue to pray for them, remembering that I once thought just like they do, and that, when it comes to diet, if I could change, anyone can.

Then there are people like my brother who say, "You were sick. You *had* to change. When I get sick, I'll change, too."

My response is always the same: "Why wait until you get sick? Why not change now so you *don't* get sick? It's much easier to make the change when you are at your strongest, not at your weakest."

Sometimes the job might be an issue. I do understand the need to work and make a living. If you truly enjoy your job and your life, I don't expect or even suggest you change; however, I tell everyone, no matter how well you eat, if you are going to a job every day you do not enjoy, your health will suffer big time. The ideal situation would be to do what you love for a living while at the same time being able to eat healthfully. There should be no other answer!

We live in a world today that is so far from understanding the connection between health and diet. People's priorities are completely skewed. I know people who make over $100,000 a year but have no time to invest in learning how to eat well. We must change our ways, and it starts with our thinking. There is nothing wrong with making $100,000 a year or owning a big house, but if you are doing it at the cost of your energy and your health, it's time to reconsider your priorities.

So my reaction to people's reaction is not controlled by *their* reaction. If we look at the word "re-action," we can see that it means we changed our actions based on the situation. Before you read this book, you didn't have the information presented within. I pray but don't expect everyone who reads this book to follow the Daylight Diet, but if I can just get you to rethink some of the choices you have made and take a new action, one that will support your health, then this book was successful.

Explaining yourself

One of the questions I get most often is, how does someone adapt the Daylight Diet without being considered a social outcast? I thought when I first started eating better many years ago that this was going to be an issue for me as well, but to my pleasant surprise, I have found it to be very easy.

Like any change, at first it can be a challenge, especially when most of the world doesn't understand the reason for the change or anything about it. The raw diet is different from any other way of eating. It is becoming the new "in" thing, so it is not as challenging to be accepted today as it was just a few years ago. However, whenever anyone makes a change in his diet, not only is it weird or different to the person making the change, but the response from friends and family can be difficult to deal with. You may even start to doubt yourself if several friends and members of your family question you.

For example, if one person tells you he thinks you look under the weather, you might say to him, "How do you know how I feel?" But if 100 people came up to you that day and told you that you looked under the weather, you would probably to start to think you really were sick. When I first started eating a Daylight Diet, many people told me how crazy I was and that I needed to eat more food.

As long as you thought out the reason and purpose for going on the Daylight Diet, and you believe it is the best diet for you, you shouldn't be bothered too much by what others say. But if you are in doubt about the diet before anyone even says anything, his or her words might take you over the edge.

Before you go on the Daylight Diet—before you make any serious decisions about your health—consider these rules:

- **Rule #1:** Don't go beyond your understanding. Do the research before changing your diet so when you get these comments, you will know you are doing the right thing.
- **Rule #2:** Make the choice yourself and not because someone else talked you into it. As long as it is your choice to change, that will help keep you strong, but if you try to change for someone else, it will be harder to stick with it when the pressure is on. Even if you have the knowledge, andyou made the choice yourself, other people's words still might make you second guess your choice to go on the Daylight Diet. We are human and we have feelings and emotions. So, then:
- **Rule #3:** Don't let your feelings override your decision. I call this "decision over emotion." It is hard to be consistent if we live according to how we *feel*. Just a few days on a Daylight Diet, many of us will *feel* the need to eat at night,

or we'll base our feelings on what other people say to us. Once we make a decision, we should stick to it. Make a promise to yourself that your faith in what you are doing is so strong that you are going to stick with it, and no one is going to talk you out of it. Of course you can make the needed adjustments along the way, but stick to your decision and stay on course!

Once you feel confident in what you are doing, how do you deal with friends, family members, and others who think you have gone over the edge? Here are some suggestions:

- **Do not be overzealous.** It's easy to believe so strongly in the message that you want to persuade everyone else, too. You and I may believe the Daylight Diet is the most healthful way to eat, but it took us a while to learn this. It's going to take other people a while, too. We have to accept all people where they are.
- **Be an example.** Let people see how great you feel and look and how much energy you have. Then they will start to ask questions. That will open the door for you to give them the answers.
- **Pray for them.** I can tell you firsthand you cannot change anyone, but by prayer, you can help everyone. The strongest thing you can do for the people you love is not to create separation in your differences, but pray that they will come to see and understand the message about healing foods and how they will improve their health. There is a great saying I once heard: "Do your best, and leave the rest up to God." I can add to that: "Pray for them, and leave the rest up to God."
- **Learn these three little words:** "My doctor said…" The most amazing advice I can give you on how to fit in socially while living the Daylight Diet is to use these magic words. No matter who it is, or where you are, these three words

will work for you. Most people will not understand the harm in eating at night; they will think you are crazy. If you tell them, "My doctor said I need to stop eating at night for a while," they can usually accept it with no problem. (You really don't have to try to find a doctor to say that. Most doctors have no idea about the benefits of eating only in the daytime, but just saying that will help other people accept you and get off your case. You are really telling the truth, because *you* are your own doctor.)

Travel

The question I get most often is how to stay on the Daylight Diet while traveling. I can honestly say this has never been an issue for me, because you can get fruits and vegetables everywhere, and, as long as I plan, I usually have no problem sticking to my schedule of eating only during daytime hours.

If there does come a time I cannot, I'd usually rather skip a meal than eat when it's dark outside. But there are situations that may come up that you didn't plan for, so if you find yourself in a situation, and you choose to eat, that's OK; it's what you decide to do most of the time that counts. Remember, you don't want to put too much pressure on yourself, and you do not need to be 100 percent perfect.

On the other hand, you don't want to say things like, "I'm going on vacation, so for this trip I'm going to overindulge." That's not what I mean. What I mean is if my plane is delayed, and I am stuck in an airport and get home late and didn't eat all day, I'd choose to skip the meal and go to sleep, but you may choose to eat. If you do, that's an unplanned event that you adjusted to. There's a difference between eating late in that situation versus making a pre-planned time to "go off" the Daylight Diet.

Dating

A friend of mine, a single guy in New York City, told me it would be impossible to date while not eating at night. That thinking is the problem right there. We live our lives around nighttime eating. We let food control our schedule. We need to let our schedule control our eating times, not the other way around. You do not need to eat at nighttime ever!

Depending on the type of person you are looking to meet, it should be no problem explaining your diet to a potential date. Of course, if you are looking to date someone who really doesn't care much about health, who smokes, drinks, and enjoys late night bars, I agree; the Daylight Diet may mess up your plans. But if you really were interested in the Daylight Diet, most likely that kind of date would not be for you anyway.

There are many activities you can enjoy at nighttime that do not revolve around food: bowling, pool, an amusement park, movies. Even better advice is to find a person interested in being healthy. If you present the Daylight Diet in the right way, the person may be excited to attempt it with you.

Instead of a late night dinner, how about a sunrise picnic on the beach or at a park? If the person is into fitness, how about meeting at the gym in the morning for a workout or game of paddleball? Or a nice walk in the park in the morning or at lunchtime?

Dating in the daylight will certainly be a twist to the usual "let's go out to eat tonight." Who knows? Your date may just find your new and different approach fresh and more appealing than the norm.

If you are the type of person who enjoys the nightlife, the clubs, bars, the Daylight Diet may not work for you or your date. However, if you really are interested in getting healthy, don't let the idea that you wouldn't be able to date get in the way of a more healthful lifestyle.

Friends

Another common issue is, how do we deal with our friends and family if we are not eating at nighttime? Of course, many social events take place, and people gather over food. You can certainly be there but not eat.

A big concern with many people who are into health is, how can they go out to eat with people who are not concerned about eating right? Instead of figuring out the solution, how about going wherever they want to go and just not eat? It may seem weird at first, but eventually they will either get used to it, or if it bothers them, they will plan nonfood events. Either way, you do not have to cave in. Sip some water, or have some tea while everyone is eating. It's really not a big deal if you don't make a big deal out of it. If people are still not convinced, just tell them you ate too much during the day, and you are full, or maybe, "my doctor said..."

There are so many activities that take place around food. If you go to a ballgame or out for a walk, you do not have to grab something to eat. If people are really your friends, not eating is not going to keep them away.

Think for a moment about people who drink but make a wise decision to stop. They can still choose to spend time with their friends who occasionally have a small drink, but they will no longer feel comfortable around people who drink a lot. They would not want to get tempted, and they would also no longer see the fun or any wisdom in spending time with these people. What I am saying is, not eating when you go out with friends may end up bothering you more than it does them. The issue may not just be that they do not want to spend time with you, but that you no longer want to spend time with them. You may decide to find more like-minded friends, and that wouldn't be a bad thing.

I'm not suggesting you give up your lifelong friendships over a diet difference. That would not be wise. I'm also not comparing eating at night to getting drunk, but we need to put things in perspective.

I am married, so I do not need to worry about dating. But when I go out with my wife, if it is at nighttime, she knows I'm not going to eat. We have an unspoken rule when it comes to diet: If I don't tell her what and how to eat, she doesn't tell me. This rule would work great with friends. No one should ever let food get in the way of a relationship.

Anyone in the raw food or vegetarian movements has heard someone say at least once something crazy like, "I'm never going to date a person who eats meat," or "I'm not going to spend time with people who eat this or that."

As for me, I'm not going to let food get in the way of my relationships. However, I personally have come to enjoy being out as much as possible during the daylight hours, especially at sunrise. For this reason, when it is dark outside, if I can help it, I'd rather be home getting ready for bed.

Family

After you decide to go on the Daylight Diet, one of your biggest challenges will be getting your family to go along for the ride. Understand that most people do not eat for health. They eat for taste. If you are making food for your family, don't give them a health lesson with the meal. Just make the food taste great, and they will enjoy it.

In my family, when I was growing up, we each had different eating times and never made it a point to sit down at the table together. So that was simple. What if your family is used to sitting down and enjoying dinner together? You can still sit down at the same time you usually do; it just doesn't have to be over food. Your conversation may be even more interesting if you are not throwing food down your mouth. If you really feel it's necessary to eat with the family, and you can't manage a midday meal, maybe everyone can get together for breakfast before leaving the house in the morning. If you are getting up early, there should be time for this.

PART IV

Achieving The Daylight Diet

CHAPTER 18

TAKE TIME TO SCHEDULE.

Planning is crucial for success.

If you've ever been in debt, you know you have to develop a budget and stick with it to get out of debt. Then, you have to do things differently to avoid going back into debt, because, if you keep doing things the way you did them before, you'll be right back where you started. So you keep that budget, that plan, and you don't deviate from it.

Likewise, I always needed a plan when I was working out at the gym. I always loved working out for my chest and arms, but not my legs, so I learned early to follow a schedule. Otherwise, I'd have ignored my legs and would quickly have become out of balance. A schedule keeps things in order.

Understanding and planning how to use your time and energy are the keys to success when you are improving your health with the Daylight Diet. Because we are in a habit of doing things a certain way, we may feel like doing this differently from what our schedule indicates we should be doing.

I've learned with my finances and with my exercise program that a schedule is what determines discipline. The lack of energy and the lack of a schedule can make the Daylight Diet almost impossible for you to follow. The energy part is easy: once we start eating according to the Daylight Diet, we automatically start absorbing more nutrients and use less energy than we are expending. The timing of our meals, however, is crucial: you cannot be successful at the diet without being on a schedule; meals must be taken at the correct times or close to them. You must create a time schedule and stick to it. If your plan is to eat your first meal at 8 a.m., you can't stay in bed until 10 a.m. Your whole day will be off schedule if you don't start at the right time.

When planning your schedule, it helps to detach yourself from your emotions. You won't plan your meals correctly if you panic when you realize you have to be up at sunrise in order to get breakfast in time to leave for work—especially if you're not used to getting up that early. If you're having negative emotional responses as you plan, you'll probably fudge a little on the times. While you don't need to follow the plan to the exact second, the farther off schedule you get, the greater the chance of failing. The more you get used to a schedule, though, the easier it will be to stick with the plan. It *will* become routine, trust me.

Early to bed

Your biggest problem at first will be getting to sleep on time. If you go to bed too late, you'll probably oversleep in the morning. But it's not only harmful things that can throw you off track. Sometimes exciting, good things can also mess up your schedule so be wary of those, too. For example, I've been on the diet for a while now, but even now as I'm writing this book, I'm tempted to stay up and write late into the night and until the wee hours of the morning.

If I weren't on a schedule, this temptation would overtake me quickly. If that were the case, I would stay up very late into the night. Not only would I not get my best writing done, the next day I would be tired, stressed, rushed, and worst of all, off schedule. Without a doubt, the best time for me to write is very early is the morning after a good night's sleep. My thinking is fresh, my excitement is high, and I'm not bothered with phone calls or rushed because it's late in the day.

Whenever I am off schedule with my diet or sleeping times, I find I am either sleeping too little or too much; but when I am on schedule, I sleep around eight hours, and usually I feel great the next day. Some people may need only seven hours, and some may need nine; right now, I do my best on eight. Of course, I can get by with far less sleep and survive, but the goal is to thrive, not just survive. How much sleep we need each night varies for each person, but, in general, most people do not get enough sleep. From a health and healing standpoint, when the body is sleeping, it is healing. A sick person needs to sleep more. Some sick people may even require 10 to 12 hours a night.

The best time to get to sleep is a question I get often. It is very common to work a 9 to 5 job in today's world. That's eight hours. Taking into consideration that people have to work and cannot get to bed as early as sunset, and that they usually need eight hours a night, I am convinced that best time to sleep seems to be 9 p.m. to 5 a.m. This is feasible if we are on the Daylight Diet and don't watch late-night television or schedule our life around late-night activities. In today's world, 10 p.m. to 6 a.m. may be more realistic, but the more hours before midnight the better. Any later than that puts your health at risk.

In the wintertime, when the days are shorter and nights are longer, we require more sleep. This is another great example of how the divine schedule works. Because foods in the winter months are heavier and take more energy to digest, so we need more sleep. In the summertime, foods are lighter and easier to digest. The days are longer, and we need less sleep.

In cases where people may require much more sleep than just eight or nine hours, the body may really need the rest, but that should not keep a person from eating the Daylight Diet. There will be no quicker way to heal than to stop eating at nighttime. In these cases, until healing has taken place and a person has recovered, it would be wise to get to sleep as early as possible so you are getting up with the sun or at least early in the morning. This would keep you on schedule.

I believe anyone can create a schedule that fits his or her situation while eating and living according to the Daylight Diet. If you feel you need more sleep than eight or nine hours a night, get to sleep earlier instead of waking up later. Extreme measures must be taken to overcome extreme situations. If you require as much as 12 hours of sleep each night, get to sleep around 6 p.m. or 7 p.m.This may seem impossibly early, but good quality sleep is needed, and you are going to get much better quality sleep getting to bed earlier. If your job or activities are in the way of getting to bed so early, rethink your schedule. Something either now or in the past has put you in a situation where you need a lot of sleep. Chances are your lifestyle needs to change. I suggest you read my book *The Formula for Health* to get an understanding and figure out a new plan.

People often stay up late into the night believing it is best go to sleep when we feel super tired. Usually, when you are on a schedule that goes along with nature, and you are not involved in stimulating activities, you will naturally and easily get tired and fall asleep several hours before midnight.

Creating a time schedule is vital to succeeding at the Daylight Diet. But you don't have to follow my schedule. Use the sun and the moon as your guide. Look at the next day's sunrise and sunset times, and figure out the optimal times for you. (See Chapter 9 for help.)

To begin, I suggest you get to bed at a time where you get the amount of sleep you need, not just what you can get by on. And plan your day to start and end around the same time every day. So, for example, if you require eight hours of sleep and the sun comes up at 7 a.m., you want to be asleep by 11 p.m. at the latest. Even that is not ideal because it is only one hour before midnight, and the more hours before midnight you go to sleep, the better; but you must get to bed by 11 p.m. if you want to rise with the sun and still get your eight hours of sleep.

Awakening before sunrise is desirable but not necessary to achieve the Daylight Diet. However, I will say this one more time because it is so vital: the later you get up after sunrise, the more challenging the Daylight Diet will be. Remember the two rules for sleep: Get to bed before midnight, the more hours the better, and get up before or at sunrise. So even if the sun will rise at 8 a.m., it would still be wise to get to sleep before midnight. And sleeping from 9 p.m. to 5 a.m., or 10 p.m. to 6 a.m., would be ideal. Also, remember, usually more sleep is needed in the winter months when the days are shorter and the nights are longer.

When to exercise

The best time to exercise is in the morning once it's light outside, but it is not a good idea to just jump right out of bed and onto the treadmill. That is a mistake I made for many years. Even if it is light outside, it's still wise to give your body some time to wake up before it's stimulated with intense exercise, so keep that in mind when planning your schedule. You don't have to exercise in the morning, but I find that, as the day gets busy, if you don't get your exercise in early you are more than likely to just not do it. Exercising in the afternoon is fine, too, but exercising too late in the day can negatively affect your sleep.

Another advantage of the Daylight Diet is that, when you are eating and sleeping on schedule, you don't need intense exercise. Intense exercise is also stimulating, and even though it makes you feel good, it can lead to adrenal exhaustion, especially right after waking. So, get up with the sun, do some light exercises, a short run, walk, pushups, some weights, rebounding, whatever you decide, if you are in good shape and on the diet, you should not need as many hours of exercise as unhealthy people require.

So now you have the keys to plan a schedule that works best for you. Once you have your meal times, sleeping times, exercise times, or whatever else you may need to get done, next fill in your activities between those times. For some of you it may be work: for others it may be taking care of the kids, but now you have a schedule to follow.

And just before bed each night, remember to check for sunrise and sunset times so you can plan your schedule and your meals. Jot it down, and fill in the blanks with your activities for the day.

When you write it down on paper and see it, it all becomes so much clearer and easier to follow. Something like this:

> Friday, January 16th:
> Sunrise 6 a.m.; wake at 6 a.m.
> Exercise at 7 a.m.
> First meal at 8 a.m.
> Second meal at 2 p.m.
> Go to bed at 10 p.m.

CHAPTER 19

THE DAYLIGHT DIET PROGRAM

The three stages to health

Some people find they can decide to adopt the Daylight Diet tomorrow and that's it: they're there. Right out of the gate, they are getting up at sunrise, eating only raw, organic foods in two meals a day, at the ideal times, and going to bed by 9 p.m. Some of us, however, need to approach the Daylight Diet in smaller steps; so in this chapter, I provide a three-stage program for moving into the Daylight Diet.

Stage 1 gets you started, eating as much as you want but only during daylight hours. Stage 2 takes the diet to the next level, still eating as much food as you want but only during the hours of 8 a.m. and 5 p.m. Finally, Stage 3 has you eating just two or three meals a day and still only between 8 a.m. and 5 p.m. Through each stage, you also progress to the right diet—raw, ripe, fresh, organic fruits, vegetables, nuts and seeds—and go to bed and wake up at the right times.

The amount of time you stay in each stage is completely your choice. I suggest deciding how long you should stay on the first few levels by your understanding, comfort, confidence, and joy. Some of you may feel comfortable sticking to Stage 1 longer, while others move more quickly to Stage 2 or 3. Just do not get so comfortable in a stage that you don't want to take the next step. Remember, it's your choice. Do not let anyone tell you what to do, how to eat, and/or when to eat. Move to the next stage when you are ready.

If you are a parent, it is your duty to bring your child up in a healthful way. Following any stage of this plan will be much better than what most other children are taught, and your child will be much healthier because of it. Also, you will be teaching your child a lifelong lesson about healthful eating that is often missing among today's children.

Stage 1

This first stage is a simple and easy way to start the Daylight Diet. There is only one major rule: Eat only when it is daylight.

Getting in the habit of not eating when it is dark outside is what Stage 1 is all about. During this stage, eat as much as you need (within limits) during the daylight so you won't feel hungry when it is dark outside. This stage is about convincing yourself it is possible to do this, and you want to break the habit of eating once the sun goes down.

Stage 1 is not an excuse to overindulge in food when it is light outside; no matter what times of day you're eating. Small meals are always best for digestion and overall health. Realizing that, if you are feeling the urge for food when it is dark outside, you may need to eat a little more during your daytime meals. Also, at any point during this stage, if you do feel hungry when it's dark outside, have some herbal tea, lemonade (no sugar—use stevia), or fresh, strained, green vegetable juice.

By this point in the book, I hope you're convinced that it's not wise to eat when it's dark outside. If you're still in doubt, try this stage for several days—perhaps during the week, taking the weekend off—and take note of how much better you're sleeping and how much better you feel the next day.

Anyone who gives Stage 1 a fair trial should feel better over time as the body becomes cleaner and healthier. When this happens, it's time to move to Stage 2. But first, let's recap Stage 1:

- Eat enough food to keep you satisfied, but only when it's light outside.
- Try not to eat right before going to sleep even if it is still light outside.

- Improve the quality of the food you eat. Avoid processed food. Eat more fresh food.
- Go to sleep by 10 p.m. and get up at sunrise. (If this isn't enough sleep, try to go to bed earlier instead of sleeping later in the morning.)
- Avoid stimulating activities at night, such as exercise, TV, loud music, and working or playing on the computer.
- Learn what helps you relax: classical music, reading a nice book, going for a walk, etc.

Stage 2

In Stage 2, you can continue to eat as much as you need to, but only between the hours of 8 a.m. and 5 p.m. Continuing to eat fresher foods and avoiding the processed junk will be a big help, because you won't be as hungry when your body is getting the nutrients it needs.

During this stage, eat as much as you need (within limits) so you won't feel hungry after 5 p.m.This stage is about convincing yourself it is possible to do this, and you don't want to struggle with hunger at nighttime. It is best to keep the eating times the same each day, even though during this stage you may be eating more than usual during the day to avoid getting hungry at night.

Only you can decide how much food can keep you satisfied throughout the day and night. We usually think we need a lot more than we really do. So, once you figure out how much you think you need, keep trying to eat a little less and see if that works. In most circumstances, the less food, the better.

Another thing: It's time to stop this crazy practice of "naming" meals as breakfast, brunch, lunch, dinner, supper, or snacks. Don't personalize your food by giving it a name. From now on, you should call your food your "first meal of the day," your "second meal of the day," etc. This will also remind you how often you used to eat. Including brunch and snacking and everything else, most people are eating 9 and 10 meals a day.

Another big help is to drink at least four cups of water upon rising and four between meals for a total of at least eight glasses a day. Never drink water with your meals because it slows digestion.

Again, if you feel hungry after 5 p.m., it's fine to enjoy a cup of herbal tea or natural lemonade or water, but that's all.

At this stage, if you are not doing so already, add some type of exercise to your schedule. It doesn't have to be intense, but engage in some sort of activity.

When you feel comfortable at this stage, and you are not getting urges to eat at night, you are ready to move to Stage 3.

Let's recap Stage 2:

- Eat as much as you need to (within limits) but only between 8 a.m. and 5 p.m.
- Continue with Stage 1 sleeping.
- Drink at least eight glasses of water throughout the day. Four of those should be taken upon rising.
- Start an exercise program.
- Start referring to your meals as "my first meal of the day," "my second meal of the day," etc.

Stage 3

By the end of Stage 3, you will be on the total Daylight Diet program, eating only two or three meals a day and only between 8 a.m. and 5 p.m. Your food will be fresh, raw, ripe, organic fruits, vegetables, nuts, and seeds, and you will not eat or exercise when it is dark outside. At this stage, you should never have to utter, "My fourth meal of the day." Three should be the max.

Once you reach Stage 3, you may actually find you don't like to eat after dark. The only things you need to do differently in Stage 3 is to make sure all the food you're eating is fresh and that you're no longer eating foods from bags, boxes, cans, containers, and bottles. Having the highest quality foods, drinking a good amount of water upon rising and between meals, eating only two times a day (three if you feel you must) and getting to sleep well before midnight comprises the final stage of the Daylight Diet. (Some people find success eating three meals a day in the summer when the days are longer and food is lighter, and two in the winter when days are shorter and food is heavier.)

Ideally, you should have your first meal during the third hour of daylight and your last meal during the ninth hour of daylight. (See Chapter 9.) However, if you do decide to consume three meals a day, space out your meal times so that there is an equal amount of time between each meal. For example, if you are eating two meals a day and find you are waking at 6 a.m. and eating your first meal around 8 a.m., your second meal should be taken at 2 p.m. If you are eating three meals a day and getting up at the same time, you would eat at 7 a.m., 11:00 a.m., and 3 p.m. Knowing in advance that you won't eat after 5 p.m. should help you figure out what times work best.

Meals should not be large. The stomach is supposed to be the size of your fist, and the key to good digestion is not making it work so hard. Eating too much, even if you're eating two meals a day, will defeat the purpose of the Daylight Diet. The exact amount in each meal will vary based on many things, such as age, weight, lifestyle, job, and activity level, but you should always feel good after each meal. You should never feel too full or tired. If you do, you have eaten too much. A good rule is to stop eating before you feel completely full. If you are not sure when that moment is, keep in mind, as long as the food is high quality, it is much wiser to eat too little than too much. As you continue to progress with this new way of eating, you will soon be able to figure out what amount is best for you.

It is wise during Stage 3 to start limiting your herbal tea or lemonade in the evenings or better yet, do not have any at least two to three hours before going to sleep. This will assure you get the best quality, deep sleep you require. If you are drinking a sufficient amount of liquid throughout the day, there should be no need for more within two or three hours of going to sleep.

During Stage 3, you will notice your body getting rid of toxins more quickly and more efficiently than ever before. It is wise to assist your body by helping the process. Familiarize yourself with some cleansing methods, such as enemas, colonics, skin brushing, herbal cleanses, and infrared saunas. They will assist you during every stage of the Daylight Diet but are essential during Stage 3. I have some excellent books at my website www.rawlife.com on these topics, and you can also find a bunch of information on the Internet.

Let's recap Stage 3:

- Your diet should consist of raw, ripe, fresh, organic fruits, vegetables, nuts, and seeds.
- Eat two meals a day, three at most.
- Eat only at the third and ninth hours of daylight if possible, but not before 8 a.m. or after 5 p.m.
- Stop intake of liquids no later than two hours before going to sleep.
- Introduce other methods of cleansing, such as infrared saunas, colonics, enemas, and skin brushing.

And that's it.

There you have the Daylight Diet plan, the ideal eating program all laid out for you. Remember, you do not have to get it right to the exact second every day 100 percent of the time. Don't make it too stressful. That will defeat the purpose and shatter the goal.

Things to consider besides what and when to eat are the mental aspects, environmental conditions, travel schedule, people around you, work, etc. All these factors should be considered to come up with the best plan for you. Do not let these situations control you and keep you from achieving your goal, but use them with wisdom to make a realistic plan that you will enjoy. Remember, you can adjust your plan as much as you need to until it fits exactly with what works best for you.

There is one more thing you should do: have fun, and enjoy the ride!

One meal a day?

You can take the Daylight Diet even further and try eating only one meal a day. Most people who do this, however, find that they eat too much food in that one meal and create more damage than good.

I don't really see the need to eat only one meal a day. Two meals a day is a very reasonable goal that we can all accomplish with ease once we understand and complete Stages 1 and 2.

Some of you may decide not to stay on Stage 3 after giving it a try. Although not ideal, eating according to Stages 1 and 2 is still better than eating when dark outside.

CHAPTER 20

MONITORING YOUR HEALTH

How to tell if you're really healthy

Most people decide if something is working or not based on how they feel, yet feelings aren't always the accurate way to monitor progress.

How you feel will usually be a result of what your body has adapted to, not what's really going on. Take a smoker, for instance. Someone who has been smoking two packs of cigarettes for many years can do so without coughing. But a person who's never smoked will cough. If you were "listening to your body" or deciding things by how you feel, in this example you would think the person who doesn't cough has the stronger lungs and that it's OK for them to smoke because it doesn't appear that smoking makes them "feel" bad. We all realize that would be crazy reasoning, but that's exactly what people do when they decide their health by how they "feel."

Don't get me wrong. How you feel should always be figured into the equation, because, no matter what you are doing, if you do not feel good or great, something may not be working for you. Feeling great on a consistent basis is usually a good indicator you are doing things right, but this is not always the case. Unless you have been eating the Daylight Diet for many years, your body probably isn't yet at the point where it has completely cleansed and healed itself, and it may not be able to give a true picture of what is really happening on the inside.

Several factors and views should always be used to monitor your level of health. If you look into the window of a house, you are only going to get a view of what the window reveals. You will get even more information if you look into another window. The body works the same way. There are several ways to tell what is going on inside the body and taking advantage of as many ways as possible will benefit you the most. The more views we have to help us monitor our level of health, the better.

Three important ways to monitor our health include the quality of our digestion, sleep, and blood. These three things work synergistically; so never give less attention to one than the other. All three must be used together to get the best answers.

Digestion

Years ago, when I was writing my first book, *The Raw Life*, I interviewed colon therapist Gil Jacobs. He told me you can tell everything about your health by your bowel habits. I find that to be excellent advice. Do you go to the bathroom several times a day or are you constipated? When you do go, is it comfortable or painful? Do you have gas throughout the day? All of these are reflections of your level of health.

Good digestion equals good health. Regardless of how you "feel," if your digestive system is not working well, you are not in good health. If your digestion is working as it should, you will notice you go to the bathroom every day.

My own illness (IBD) happened because I ignored what my body needed, and I didn't pay attention to my digestion. If I would have just paid attention to the digestive process, I would have figured out I was doing something wrong long before I was seriously ill and at a later stage of disease.

We all have this great opportunity to pay attention and react to the signs of the body long before we experience the consequences of ignoring them. Simply learn and pay attention; then react accordingly. Soon, you'll realize when your body is screaming at you to control your eating habits.

Fortunately, you do not need to wait until that point. You do not need to be diagnosed with inflammatory bowel disease or colon cancer before you figure out your digestive system is not doing its job. Simply monitor your bowel movements, pay attention to any gas you may have, and look at your stomach in the mirror. Do you have gas often? Does your stomach stick out? Do you have easy, pain-free bowel movements every day?

Your answers reveal more about your health than you think. Correcting digestive problems begins with the Daylight Diet.

Chews to chew

The amount of food, number of meals, quality of food, and times you eat all affect digestion, but there is more that needs to be done to keep your digestive system working well. After we swallow, the food we've eaten is more or less out of our control. Before that, though, we have total control. Proper mastication and food combining can prevent many digestive problems.

Digestion begins in the mouth. Saliva contains an enzyme that helps break down the food and jump-starts digestion. Chewing helps the body more readily extract the nutrients from the food and cuts down on the work the digestive system has to do. The less work the digestive tract has to do, the more efficiently it will do its job. When we don't chew our food well, it can ferment in our digestive system. The more food is chewed, the easier it is to digest, and the healthier it will be for the body. Even raw foods can cause problems if they're not properly chewed.

Eating less food seems impossible to some people because they do not chew their food well, and the nutrients are not completely absorbed. This leaves the person unsatisfied, the cells deficient, and the whole system of the body out of order.

The reason we shouldn't drink water or any liquids with our meals is because they dilute the digestive effects of the saliva. Drink water and liquids between meals, not with meals.

Food combining

The order in which we eat our food, called sequential eating, and the types of food we eat together, called food combining, play a big role in good digestion. Eating the wrong foods together or in the wrong order can sap our energy and cause fermentation and putrefaction in the digestive system.

Food combining and sequential eating allow for easier digestion and minimal digestive conflicts. It works like this: Every food takes a certain amount of time to digest. Eating similar foods with similar digestive times helps the body digest meals more easily; these foods are said to combine well. For example, watermelon takes about one hour to digest; almonds may take up to five hours. In view of this, eating watermelon and almonds at the same meal is not a good idea, so it's known as a poor combination. Eating too many meals like this may cause constipation, bloating, and gas, which may lead to more serious issues.

Since there are different types of raw food, each with its own unique digestive time, your body will have to work harder to digest foods eaten in poor combinations. Ideally, your body will use as little energy as possible for digestion—the very reason it's important to combine your foods properly. In general, it helps to eat high liquid foods with other high liquid foods and dense foods with other dense foods.

Sequential eating is similar to food combining, but instead of combinations, sequential eating focuses on consuming one food at a time. It advocates eating the most easily digested foods first and denser foods last. (I offer several books on my website to explain food combining: www.rawlife.com. To learn more about sequential eating, visit www.drbass.com.)

Most people know little or nothing about food combining and sequential eating. The average person has never heard that the order in which we eat food can play a big part in digestion and health. People often tell me they have tried a raw food diet and that it didn't work for them. My answer is always, if you don't understand *how* to eat your food, you can make your health problems worse.

Take a deep breath.

Deep breathing and clean air also are essential to good digestion and overall health. Pure, fresh air helps the blood circulate more easily throughout the body and helps the organs work to their best capability.

Deep breathing supplies the blood with oxygen. Each breath exhaled releases carbon dioxide that, if not released from the body, can become toxic, resulting in poor digestion and other health issues.

Here's what Dr. Dio Lewis has to say about the important role the digestive system plays in good health, from his 1870 book, *Talks about People's Stomachs:*

> "One reason for the marked constitutional disturbance which comes of stomach trouble is that we have only one stomach, and when that fails, the whole body must fail. Now one lung may fail and the other go on well. I have known many such cases. A former patient of mine, now residing in Washington, has not taken a breath into his right lung in many years, and yet in an important public position, he works better than the average. Of course his body is not vigorous, for his breathing is insufficient; still he has a comfortable, healthy life and is doing good service.
>
> "The brain is in two halves; one may retire from active service and the other go on. We have two legs, two arms, and two eyes. We may lose one and not get off the track. But we have only one stomach, and if that gets off the track, the whole man is knocked into a heap."

Sleep

No matter how good you may feel, if you are not getting the proper amount of sleep your body needs, your overall health and wellness will be negatively affected.

A recent survey found that more people are sleeping less than six hours a night, and three-quarters of us have problems sleeping at least a few nights a week. Failing to get enough sleep or sleeping at odd hours heightens the risk for a variety of major illnesses, including cancer, heart disease, diabetes, and obesity, not to mention decreased performance and alertness, impaired memory and cognition and increased stress.

The exact amount of sleep each person needs may vary, but if you don't get what you need on a nightly basis, you can't stay healthy for long. Sometimes you may not even know you didn't get a good night's sleep unless you feel tired the next morning.

How we feel often is the result of how well we slept the night before, but on a long-term basis, one good night's worth of sleep does not erase many days and weeks of an unhealthy, inconsistent sleeping pattern. Not getting enough sleep goes directly against the Daylight Diet program. It's nearly impossible to go to sleep at odd hours each night and under sleep and then expect to be successful at the Daylight Diet. In fact, no matter what diet you are eating, good, consistent rest is essential.

We quickly forget how much we slept the night before, or two nights before, or last week. To monitor your sleep, keep a sleep log. That way, you can look over it in a week or two and know exactly whether the way you feel relates to how well or how long you have been sleeping.

Not getting good quality sleep usually is directly related to diet. If I have eaten too much or too late, I certainly do not sleep as well as when I strictly follow the Daylight Diet.

Blood

> There are two paths; one is leading to life, and the other is to death. If you don't know which path you are on, that's choosing death. Life is a commitment! Choose life! — **Dr. Emil Schandl**

Blood tests detect abnormalities that may lead to serious diseases years before a possible, tragic diagnosis.

The blood is like the messenger of the body; it reveals what is going on inside. It can even help predict the future. There are many different blood tests that can reveal a host of different answers to help you pinpoint possible issues with your diet, digestion or assimilation The sooner you find out, the sooner you can take care of it.

Years ago, I was feeling great but decided to check my blood anyway. I was surprised to find, though my blood was good, I still had some developing issues. There was no other way I could have uncovered those issues other than getting my blood checked. I made some adjustments in my diet and lifestyle, and everything cleared up. Now I am a big believer in monitoring my blood work every six months, and it is one of my strongest recommendations.

No matter what your health program, it's a wise idea to get your blood monitored at least once a year. I would suggest starting with a basic Complete Blood Count (CBC). It's the most common blood test, and you can get it from just about any doctor or medical office. Then get tested for everything your insurance will cover, such as B-12 and vitamin D. (Neither of these tests is part of a CBC.)

My friend Dr. Schandl, a biologist, a clinical chemist, and a nutritional consultant, has created a compressive list of blood tests he calls the Longevity Blood Profile© and Cancer Profile© to help people monitor just about every aspect of their health. I suggest visiting his website and leaning more about what test he has to offer. (www.caprofile.net)

If the CBC indicates anything out of range, I would suggest you take other related tests, even if insurance won't cover it. Since most nutrients work synergistically, getting a good variety of tests will be the best choice. Don't worry; you do not need to be a whiz to figure it all out. Any good nutritionist can advise you on the matter.

Monitoring your blood and paying attention to your bowel habits and sleep patterns can help you figure out exactly what's going on with your health. These things are important to know, because, even though you may feel great, damage can be taking place.

Navel gazing

Finally, there is one more way to monitor your health. Take off your shirt, and look at your stomach. Do you have a gut sticking out? A little or a lot? Perhaps it's sticking out beyond your chest. If it's sticking out at all, it's a good sign you are not eating well, and, as a result, you are bloated or have excess fat or gas around your waist.

Another sign you may not be well is if you have gas. That is a common sign fermentation is going on inside the body as a result of unhealthful eating.

Use all these signs to monitor your health more accurately.

CHAPTER 21

GOOD COUNSEL

Whom to turn to

It is my sincere prayer that, if you made it this far into the book, you are either already eating a Daylight Diet, or you have been motivated to start very soon. I want to assist you in the process, making it as simple as possible for you and your body. The best way I know how to do that is to give you tips and suggestions that have helped me and many others in the past.

I can think of no better way to get on the right track and stay there than by having the advice of an experienced person to help you. We can all learn from our mistakes, of course, but why do so if you don't have to? Not eating at nighttime is a great way to improve your overall health, but there is even more you can do. Get good guidance.

Once you find the right person to help coach you on the path, the more information you can supply them with the better. People who are already dealing with some kind of health issue often contact me, and when they come to me with a lot of information, it's easier and quicker for me to put together a program that works best for them. However, the sad fact is that usually people do not have much information other than they "don't feel good," or "the doctor said this."

You need more information than that to pinpoint issues and come up with the best plan. Here is what I suggest to people who are serious about their health:

1. Get an exam by a doctor.

I don't always suggest people go visit a doctor, and I rarely suggest anyone listen to a doctor, but if something is wrong with your health, getting a diagnosis by a doctor can be the first step in creating a natural healing for yourself. I meet people who say they never need to go to a doctor. Sometimes it can really help. Let me give you an example.

Someone calls me on the phone and is concerned because he has blood in the stool when going to the bathroom. I ask what the issue is, but, other than the blood and some pain, the person doesn't know. There could be any of a number of things wrong, from a minor hemorrhoid to a tumor or something in between. Often it is IBD, and it's why I am being contacted, but for me to really help, I need to know all the issues.

In most cases, an adjustment in diet and lifestyle will be all that's needed to help, but, in more serious cases, much more cleansing and certain herbs and other therapies must be included. Remember, this is your health, so you don't want to take chances. In every case, a Daylight Diet will help the problem.

Not everyone has a major issue. People just want to improve their health and prevent any major issues from happening, so not everyone needs to go visit a doctor. But if you have a consistent pain, bleeding, swelling, or lump, or often feel dizzy or notice anything else that is becoming different from the norm and is bothering you, visiting a doctor would be wise. Doctors do not always diagnose correctly; however, they have access to machines, technology, and tests that can help rule out many conditions and help pinpoint problems.

2. Get extensive blood tests or at least a Complete Blood Count (CBC).

The importance and types of blood work were discussed in Chapter 20. I recommend blood tests for everyone. I can give basics about diet, but to really help, it's best to know what the blood work reveals. Even if you choose not to get the full profiles, a basic CBC can indicate a lot about what's happening in the body.

3. See a nutritional consultant.

Once you have all the information in Steps 1 and 2, I suggest taking that information to a good nutritional consultant. This person should have many years of experience and come highly recommended. There are many people who write books and teach, but they do not have a good understanding about the body and how our health relates to our diet. A person doesn't necessarily need to be a professional nutritional counselor, but he needs to know what he is doing. If you mention the Daylight Diet, and he disagrees, I would make a quick exit and find somebody else.

I occasionally do nutritional counseling, especially for people who have IBD. I love to help everyone, but because of my busy travel schedule, it's often difficult for me to find the time to do personal consultations. I can always recommend someone if I am not available, so if you cannot find anyone, visit my website www.Paulnison.com, and you can see more information there about making an appointment with me.

I am excited to help the person who want to help themselves. If someone has taken some or all of the steps I've mentioned and read my books and seen my videos, I am usually able to help people put the final pieces together to complete his or her own unique health puzzle. It's been my experience that following the Daylight Diet is the best way to deal with potential and existing health issues related to diet.

I can adjust your program, but what I am especially good at and excited about is making it easier for you and getting you motivated to do it. Making a change your eating times quickly is not that simple and often may even seem impossible. There are many emotional aspects to late-night eating, plus issues such as dealing with family and friends. After you have followed these steps, or even before, visit my website, check out my blog, and sign up for my daily newsletter. The information I share is the latest and most updated information to help you help yourself.

You can stay updated on my travel schedule to see when I will be speaking in your town, and you can also visit my blog for daily updates on new discoveries and motivational messages to help you.

CHAPTER 22

EXCEPTIONAL CIRCUMSTANCES

Is the Daylight Diet ever a bad idea?

I have said repeatedly throughout this book that *the* Daylight Diet is the solution to so many health problems and is the way everyone should eat to prevent illness. Is there ever a time when a person should *not* adopt the Daylight Diet?

The most common objection to the Daylight Diet that I hear is that people with blood sugar problems need to eat often to keep their glucose at a good level and on an even keel. Millions of people suffering from diabetes and hypoglycemia often question if they could eat so little food as the Daylight Diet suggests.

Their question shows their lack of knowledge that so many people and doctors have about these conditions. It's an unhealthful eating pattern and poor diet that has created the problem. Continuing to eat against the divine schedule and the foods that were never meant to be in our body in excess will only make the conditions worse. The real answer is to get rid of the cause of the problem, and that is exactly what the Daylight Diet will do.

There are some circumstances for which the Daylight Diet is not the best diet:

Pregnancy and breastfeeding

During the time I was writing this book, my wife gave birth to a beautiful baby girl, Noa Raquel. We decided to have a natural home birth, and we are feeding our little baby only breast milk for now. God's wonderful design lets us know the best food and times that are most natural for our newborn baby. Every three to four hours Noa must be fed. Not only is she crying for nourishment, but also my wife's breasts engorge with milk to supply

Noa with just the right amount for each feeding.

Our baby, of course, cannot and should not be on the Daylight Diet, since babies need to eat whenever they're hungry. Besides, even the name "Daylight Diet" doesn't apply, since Noa could find her mother's breast in the dark, so breastfeeding at all hours is not going against natural instincts for a baby. However, grown-ups cannot find their food in the dark, just another example of how un-natural it is to try to do so.

My wife also should not be attempting a Daylight Diet at this time. An expectant mother should not have a problem with the Daylight Diet (at least on Stage 1), but a breastfeeding momma is truly eating for two; during the first year, the mom could add one more meal to her normal Daylight Diet, even if it is at nighttime. I think it would still be wise to make sure the meal is taken before 9 p.m. There is no reason any breastfeeding mom would need to eat between the hours of 9 p.m. and morning daylight if she were eating good, nutritious food throughout the day. However, this is our first baby, and so far my wife doesn't need to eat after 9 p.m. I have heard from other moms who disagree, though, so breastfeeding moms should probably eat as much as you feel you need, whenever you feel you need to. One thing I know for sure is, you've earned it. However, as your baby grows and you stop breastfeeding, get back on the Daylight Diet.

The night shift

If you work at night, you may not be able to eat according to the Daylight Diet; however, understand that working a nighttime job goes against the divine schedule for a healthy life just as much as eating at night does. I address this in Chapter 8, but I'll say it again here: All of us make choices about where and when we work. If you value your health, you need to know that studies show that people who work the night shift are not as healthy as those who work in the daytime. That's why they call it the "graveyard" shift.

While you still work at nighttime, try to eat as much as possible when it is daylight outside, and if you must eat when it is nighttime, have that meal as close to sunrise or sunset as possible. Make sure, whatever you do, that you do not eat during the middle of the night. If you are eating two meals a day, one in the daytime and the other around sunrise or sunset should be enough.

Special events

If there is some special occasion—your daughter is getting married and dinner is served at nighttime—you do not have to refuse your meal. If eating at nighttime is only a very rare occasion, don't fret. It's OK. Plan ahead on these occasions, and try not to eat much during the day; maybe you could skip a meal and replace it with the special nighttime meal on that day.

This book is for you. If you can think of any other reason you can absolutely not eat a Daylight Diet, don't count it out completely. Make the proper adjustments, eat less food when you do eat, and enjoy everything you do (except eating at night). Above all, don't make yourself sick worrying about it.

CHAPTER 23

PUTTING IT ALL TOGETHER

There's more to it than just food.

Whenever talking about health, I cannot leave out the importance of exercise, water, sunshine, and fresh air. A book could be written on each of these topics so necessary for good health. I will do my best to give the importance of each subject justice here within this chapter. The study of these subjects needs to be clearly understood, so I encourage everyone to study these subjects further. (Join my free e-newsletter and my blog for the latest health information on these topics and more. See www.paulnison.com)

Exercise

Exercise is something people either avoid or partake of way too much; they're either overactive or couch potatoes. As I said at the beginning of this book, you must get the right amount; too little or too much can cause many healthy issues. I suggest you exercise in ways that will help every part of your body maintain its good health. The right amount of exercise aids the body in detoxifying and cleaning the lymph system and has many other important health benefits.

There are different types of exercise: cardiovascular, muscle building, balance, core, and stretching to increase flexibility. The healthier you are, the less intense exercise you need. If you are on the Daylight Diet, there is no reason to go to extreme lengths with your exercise. Just about every fitness need can be met by brisk walking, stretching, and calisthenics. There is no need to pay a lot of money to join a gym or buy exercise equipment.

Before technology encouraged our sedentary lifestyles, our

daily active lifestyles kept us fit. We would get our exercise during our daily life. We have to make fitness part of our daily routine. Walk to the store instead of driving; lift things instead of having machines do it; stretch and breathe deeply each day. Do your best to be active. (One great exercise I can think of for everyone would be to pick up your TV sets, walk them to the garbage, and throw them in the trash.) The Daylight Diet is a great start to an active lifestyle. Remember, whatever exercise you choose, make sure it is something you enjoy.

Water

In every good health book I've ever read, drinking water throughout the day is always touted for its health benefits.

Water, the simplest liquid available, is the only liquid that cleans the body and at the same time doesn't require any energy to digest. But you must make sure the water you're putting into your body is the cleanest you can get. Putting dirty water into your body will also cause problems. You wouldn't try to clean the outside of your body with soap that had dirty oil in it, so why try to clean your insides with dirty water? Drink plenty of clean water, and you will be clean and feel wonderful.

About three-quarters of the human body is composed of water, and the circulation of water throughout the body is immense. One of the great contributory causes of old age is lack of sufficient water in the system. Lack of water is also one of the greatest causes of constipation, which is the beginning of most diseases. Drinking enough water throughout the day will help wash your body out. It will give your body an inner bath.

The best time of the day to drink water is upon rising in the morning. Water will help the body rid loosened waste from the nightly cleanse and can also help the body have a smooth bowel movement. A great book I suggest everyone read is *Your Body's Many Cries for Water.* The author, Dr. F. Batmanghelidj, talks about dehydration as the main disease of people today.

Sunshine

Enjoying the sun is another important key to health that most Americans tend to avoid. Contrary to popular belief, sunshine is good for you as long as you're smart about it. As long as you don't abuse sunrays, they will never cause harm. The sun was created as a tool for our well-being. The sun supplies warm weather, nutrients, and light.

Health and happiness (and getting enough vitamin D) require exposing your skin and eyes to the sun on a regular basis. The cleaner your body becomes, the more you'll realize this. The sunlight will actually keep your skin soft and beautiful. However, no matter the state of your health, burning skin is never healthful. If you are sunburned, you've stayed in the sun too long; you've had more than enough for that day, whether it's five minutes or five hours. It's different for everyone. Do not stay out long enough to get burned. Anything short of that should be fine.

Air

Keep windows open at nighttime or sleep outside if you can. A person can live without food for weeks, without water only for days, but without air, only minutes. Clean pure oxygen is the most important thing for our survival. Diseases can only survive and become harmful when our bodies lack pure air. Because of shallow breathing and poorly ventilated houses and workplaces, people are getting sicker.

Prayer

Finally, in closing, I have found nothing heals better and relieves stress more than prayer. Having a relationship and ongoing communication with God is the best solution to all things. He designed our body and told us what to eat and when. Read my book *Health According to the Scriptures* for more information on this important topic (available at www.rawlife.com).

CONCLUSION

Time to take action

Even though this is the conclusion to this book, there is really no end to the Daylight Diet. The limits to which you can take this idea go far beyond any other diet system. It was created at the beginning of time as one of the essential elements for our well-being. As we drift away from the divine laws of the Creator, we suffer. Just as there is the law of gravity and the breath of life, some things were created for our essential existence. The Daylight Diet is another one of these essential laws we must follow if we want to be healthy.

We live in such a time of sickness and death. Man spends billions of dollars each year for an answer to disease and searches the deepest parts of the world when the real answer simply lies right in front of him—and it is free. The sun and the moon were given to us as a way to schedule our lives, our eating, and our sleep. If we use them wisely and follow the divine laws of our Creator, our capacity to live a long, healthy life is boundless.

"Old age" is a new term. People used to say instead, "long life." There is a difference between old age and a long life. Barely surviving while living out your final days in an old age home is not the same as thriving while looking young and having wonderful amounts of energy in your later stages of life. All the successful health writers I have read and spoke about confirm a moderate diet and eating at the right times are the most healthful way to get there.

As I research the health writers from the 18th and 19th Centuries, I find never is the word "cancer" mentioned. In this book, I often quote the writings of Dr. Dio Lewis from the mid-to-late 1800s and not even then are cancer or diabetes or other diseases that plague us today mentioned. Why is this? Have the sun and moon disappeared? Can they no longer guide us?

No. What has changed is people no longer pay attention to these important signs as they once did. People no longer listen to their bodies crying to them to stop the excess amounts of food and to stop eating at night. People treat their bodies as if it were objects of outward beauty, spending more time and money trying to fix the outside while ignoring the inside. They have no idea that if you take care of the inside, the outside will look fine.

Thinking about the great health advice and wisdom from writers of the past, I would suggest that before you eat something, think about whether it was considered food 100 years ago. If it wasn't, we should probably think twice about considering it food today. In addition, if we can't grow more food from the food we're putting into our mouth, we should probably limit how much of that food we put into our bodies. And finally, if it has to go through your car window to be purchased, we for sure shouldn't put *that* into our mouths.

I can only suggest people wake up and start taking responsibility for the problems they created and start working on the cure. Eat a Daylight Diet for one month, and see for yourself how excellent this plan can be for you. No more excuses. The time to change is now. Some of us know the Daylight Diet works; we have been eating this way for years with great success. Others know but just need to be reminded. The rest of us are in the dark when it comes to eating right amounts and at the right times.

Health is not a random thing that some people have and some don't. It is the result of good, healthy living! There is no other way to obtain it.

Before you read this book, you may have not known it was not healthful to eat when the sun goes down or to eat more than two or three times a day. If you have gotten this far in the book, you know it now. What are you going to choose?

At one point in my life, I didn't know I had a choice about the state of my health. As a result, as a young man who was supposed to be in the prime of his life, I was a very ill person. Now, more than 15 years later, I have more energy and health than younger men I know. The difference is that now I know I have a choice, and I'm doing something about it.

Eat right and sleep right, and you have mastered the two fundamental requirements of health and long life!

A FINAL THOUGHT

The wonderful mind of Dr. Dio Lewis

When I decided to write a book about the health benefits of the Daylight Diet, I came across the wonderful writings of Dio Lewis. Dr. Lewis had a very similar message to the one I was writing about in my book, and his information was very supportive. I discovered Dio Lewis was well known during the mid-1800s as a temperance leader, later sparking the prohibition movement in the United States. We need more men like Dr. Lewis today to stand up for what is healthy and moral. His message was temperance in all good things.. I was elated to learn Dr. Lewis was a homeopathic doctor who wrote about nutrition.

I quote Dr. Lewis frequently in my book *The Daylight Diet*, but I want people to be able to read Dr. Lewis's complete works, not just my excerpts. I toyed with the idea of reprinting his book T*alks about People's Stomachs,* but instead my friends at Health Research Books (HRB), who specialize in rare and hard-to-find books, agreed to reprint it. I offered to write a short foreword for the book, and they agreed. Now this book is available to you. (Order from www.rawlife.com.)

It is the aim of his book to show the simple and natural means by which the stomach may be kept healthy. Dio Lewis had a keen eye in looking at the facial characteristics of people. He claimed if we were to watch people, we should be able to determine the condition of their stomachs. Even though this book carries a strong health message for all of us, one cannot help but pick up the author's sense of humor. This book is about stomachs, and we all have one. Flatulence is addressed as "noises in the bowels," so perfectly described one cannot help but laugh while reading this informative chapter. According to Dr. Lewis, we can choose a "short life and a merry one," or a "long life and a merry one." From sleep to digestion, this book is a treasure trove of information and is a very sweet and informative read.

Here is Dr. Lewis's introduction to *Talks about People's Stomachs*, written in 1870:

Without health, we can enjoy no fortune, honors, or riches, and all the other advantages are useless. — **Hippocrates**

"Sitting one evening near a reservoir on the brow of a hill overlooking a European city, my companion, an eminent physician, told me this story:

"About twenty years ago, I was called early one morning, to visit, in great haste, a family at whose house I had spent the previous evening. The messenger exclaimed, 'Oh! Doctor, come as quick as possible: they are all vomiting themselves to death.'

"I jumped into my clothes, seized my stomach pump and ran. The doctors were flying in all directions. We cried out to each other. 'Poison! Poison!' and rushed on. I assure you, sir, the town was given up to the wildest excitement I have ever witnessed. All suffered with the same symptoms— vomiting, retching,thirst, and burning pain.

"At ten o'clock, the mayor called a few of us together for a moment's consultation.

"I had the honor to suggest that the poison must be in the water.

"We ran up here, and right there in the corner, just under that tree, we caught a glimpse of a large paper package, and rushing into the water, we hauled out more than ten pounds of the deadly poison, still undissolved."

"The Stomach is the reservoir from which every part of the body receives its supplies, and most of its diseases.

"Let us look out at this window.

"Do you see that man with a red nose? That is produced by a poison which comes from his reservoir.

"Notice that lady with the ugly eruption. The poison which produces that comes from her stomach, or reservoir.

"There, that fine looking gentleman with a bad limp has a big toe which is *too* big. I know him well. He insists that the moon is responsible for his gout, ashis bad attacks come on at the full of the moon. Well, I tell him that the reservoirfrom which the poison in his toe comes is somewhat like the moon in shape, and so he may not be so wide of the truth after all.

"But look at that fellow! Did you ever see such a doleful face? That man has the blues fearfully: he wishes himself dead a hundred times a day. You see, his brain must receive its supplies from his stomach. But his stomach, or reservoir furnishes not sweet, healthy chyme, but acids and poisonous gases. Of course his brain gets poison instead of food. His face tells the whole story.

"If we were to stand here and see a hundred people pass, we should be able to determine the condition of their reservoirs.

"Ah! There's a good one! What a fine skin! What a bright eye! What anelastic step! That young woman's reservoir is sending to her system nourishment,and not poison.

"It is the aim of this work to show the simple and natural means by which the stomach, or reservoir, may be kept in a sweet and healthy condition.

"It is well known that I have been busy with physiological and hygienic themes for many years, and yet I do not think that the well-read student will find in this work much that is original. I have tried, rather, to present familiar thoughts in a simple and attractive dress.

"An author's ambition may have played a part in my earlier writings, but I believe I can now say with sincerity that in this little work and in three others which will quickly follow it, I simply try to make myself useful.

"Conscious of possessing important facts and ideas which may serve my countrymen, I send out these books at the mere cost of their production and with the hope that they may meet the welcome which so many have given to my previous works."

RECIPES

NUT MILKS

ALMOND MILK DRINK

2 to 3 cups almond milk
1 tablespoon green food powder (Pure Synergy)
2 teaspoons hemp powder
1 teaspoon green powder stevia
½ teaspoon maca powder
2 teaspoons chia seeds
¼ teaspoon camu powder
¼ teaspoon sea salt
6 ice cubes

Process all of the ingredients in a blender or a food processor until completely smooth. Makes 2 servings.

HEMP MILK DRINK

1 cup water
½ cup hemp seeds
1 tablespoon maca powder
2 teaspoons raw carob powder
½ teaspoon camu powder
1 tablespoon green powder stevia
Sea salt to taste
1 tablespoon green powder
1 tablespoon chia seeds
Ice cubes

Process all of the ingredients in a blender or a food processor until completely smooth. Makes 2 servings.

"EGG" NOG

No, this is nothing like the eggnog you're familiar with: It's better!

1 vanilla bean
2 cups almond milk
1 cup macadamia nuts
1/2 cup raw honey
1 tablespoon ground cinnamon
1 teaspoon ground nutmeg
1/4 teaspoon turmeric
1 banana, cut into 4 or 5 pieces

Slice the vanilla bean in half lengthwise with the tip of a sharp knife. Scrape the seeds from each half and place into blender. Add all of the remaining ingredients to the blender. Process until smooth. Makes about 4 cups.

SALADS AND SALAD DRESSINGS

PAUL'S POWERFUL SALAD

I call this my "powerful" salad because every ingredient is a powerhouse of nutrients.

Fresh spinach leaves (as much as you like)
½ medium cucumber, chopped
½ stalk celery, chopped
1 avocado, peeled, pitted, and chopped
½ red bell pepper, cored, seeded, and chopped (optional)
1 to 2 tablespoons ground flaxseeds
Juice of 1 lemon

Place the spinach, cucumber, celery, avocado, and red bell pepper, if desired, into a large bowl. Toss together to combine. Sprinkle with flaxseeds and lemon juice. Makes 1 serving.

HERB DRESSING

This tastes great over broccoli.

2 stalks fresh fennel
½ cup fresh cilantro
1 cup walnuts
½ onion
Sea salt to taste
½ cup nutritional yeast

Process all of the ingredients in a blender or a food processor until completely smooth. Makes about 2 cups.

CAESAR DRESSING

½ cup almond butter
½ cup pine nuts
Salt to taste
Juice of ½ lemon
2 cloves garlic
Cayenne to taste

Process all of the ingredients in a blender or a food processor until completely smooth. Makes about 1 cup.

RED TAHINI

½ cup sesame seeds
2 cloves garlic
Juice from ½ lemon
½ red bell pepper
Cayenne to taste

Process all of the ingredients in a blender or a food processor until completely smooth. Makes about 1 cup.

CARROT GINGER SALAD DRESSING

5 carrots
2-inch piece fresh ginger
¼ cup water or apple cider vinegar
1 date

Process all of the ingredients in a blender or a food processor until completely smooth. Makes about 2 cups.

SESAME GINGER DRESSING

¼ cup fresh lemon juice
1 ½ inch piece fresh ginger, peeled
1/4 cup raw sesame oil or olive oil
1 large clove garlic
1 teaspoon kelp powder
Pinch cayenne

Process all of the ingredients into a blender or a food processor until completely smooth. Makes about 1/2 cup.

ALMOND GINGER DRESSING

2 cups chopped bell pepper
1 cup raw almond butter
½ cup chopped scallion
¼ cup chopped red beet
2 teaspoons chopped fresh ginger
1 clove garlic
1 ½ teaspoons kelp powder
1 cup water
1 tablespoon nama shoyu
½ tablespoon fresh lemon juice
Cayenne to taste

Process all of the ingredients in a blender or a food processor until completely smooth. Makes about 4 cups.

CHEDDAR SAUCE

1 cup raw cashews, sunflower seeds, or almonds
½ large red bell pepper
¼ cup water
2 tablespoons fresh lemon juice
2 tablespoons nutritional yeast
1 tablespoon tahini
1 ½ teaspoons sea salt
1 clove garlic

2 teaspoons onion power or 1 small slice onion or 1 tablespoon chopped green onion Process all of the ingredients in a blender or a food processor until completely smooth, adding the water a little at a time until it reaches desired consistency. Makes about 2 cups.

TOMATO BASIL DRESSING

This dressing is especially delicious in late summer, when you're assured of fresh, ripe tomatoes and basil.

2 tomatoes, cut into quarters
1 clove garlic
Juice of ½ medium lemon
1 cup fresh basil leaves

Process all of the ingredients into a blender or a food processor until completely smooth. Makes about 2 cups.

DIPS, SPREADS, AND SAUCES

RAW HEALTHY PESTO

Serve as a dip or over pasta.

2 to 4 cloves garlic
2 bunches spinach
1 bunch fresh basil
Juice of ½ medium lemon
1 cup pine nuts
½ teaspoon Celtic sea salt
½ cup olive oil

Place garlic into a food processor. Process until the garlic is well minced. Add all of the remaining ingredients and process until completely smooth. Makes 4 servings.

TOMATO SAUCE

I also like to add a chopped avocado to this and serve it with raw pasta dishes.

3 tomatoes
½ cup sun-dried tomatoes (not packed in oil)
1 clove garlic
½ tablespoon chopped fresh basil
½ tablespoon chopped fresh oregano
1 small hot pepper, such as a jalapeño or Serrano

Place all of the ingredients into a blender or a food processor. Process until completely smooth. Makes about 2 cups.

PINE NUT DIP

Pour this over a raw salad or use it as a dip for raw, fresh vegetables.

1 cup pine nuts
½ lemon
¼ teaspoon ground nutmeg
1-inch piece fresh ginger, peeled
1 clove garlic
Sea salt to taste

Place all of the ingredients into a blender or a food processor. Process until well combined. Makes 2 cups.

ONION-WALNUT PATÉ

This is great served with raw vegetables, or slice and serve as an entrée.

1 cup minced onion
¼ cup loosely packed parsley
2 cups soaked walnuts
2 teaspoons pine nuts
Sea salt to taste

Process all of the ingredients into a blender or a food processor until completely smooth. Makes 5 to 8 servings.

CHIA TAPIOCA PUDDING

¼ cup of chia seeds
1 cup almond, banana or coconut milk
2 tablespoons raw raisins
Ground cinnamon to taste

In a medium bowl, mix chia seeds and milk. Place into refrigerator for 10 minutes.

Add raisins and stir in cinnamon. Return to refrigerator overnight, stirring several times. You may need to stir once again before serving. Makes about 1 1/2 cups.

BLENDED MEALS

BLENDED SALAD

For better digestion, try drinking your salads instead of chewing them. Here's one of my favorites.

1 cup spinach or lettuce leaves
½ medium cucumber, cut into 3 or 4 pieces
1 stalk celery, cut into 3 or 4 pieces
Juice of ½ lemon
1 cup sunflower sprouts (optional)
½ red bell pepper, cored, seeded, and cut into 4 or 5 pieces (optional)
1 avocado, pitted and peeled
1 teaspoon flaxseed or olive oil (optional)
1 tomato, roughly chopped

Process all of the ingredients into a blender or a food processor until completely smooth. Makes 2 to 3 servings.

COCONUT AVOCADO DRINK

Coconut and avocado make a surprisingly good combination.

Meat and water from 1 young coconut
1 avocado, pitted and peeled

Process all of the ingredients into a blender or a food processor until completely smooth. Makes 1 serving.

COCONUT, SPINACH, AND AVOCADO DRINK

Spinach gives this unusual drink more depth of flavor.

Meat and water from 1 young coconut
1 cup spinach leaves or other greens
1 avocado, pitted, and peeled

Place the meat and water of the coconut into the blender. Process until smooth. Place the spinach and avocado into the blender with the coconut. Process again until smooth. Makes 2 cups.

ABOUT THE AUTHOR

At age 20, Paul Nison was diagnosed with inflammatory bowel disease, also known as Crohn's disease, and ulcerative colitis, a deadly affliction. His search for a cure began with medical doctors, but they didn't have the answers he needed. After trying almost every "cure" to overcome his pain and suffering, Paul finally discovered the benefits of eating more simply. Simplifying his diet was the first step in his cure.

Paul started to leave out all unhealthful foods, and the healthful foods he was left with were raw, ripe, fresh, organic fruits, vegetables, nuts, and seeds.

After turning to a simple, raw food diet, Paul was amazed at how quickly his health returned. He was even more astonished because doctors told him raw foods would not help his condition. In fact, they warned him that a diet of raw fruits and vegetables would be harmful to anyone with inflammatory bowel disease. This led Paul to simplify every area of his life.

With his new understanding of "less is more," Paul left his office job in the financial industry on Wall Street, wrote several health books and started traveling lecturing about health and living simply. He didn't know it at the time, but his return to health and a simpler lifestyle was just the beginning of a path that would bring him to question the connection between today's fast-paced, urban lifestyle with the sadly diseased state in which so many people find themselves.

Paul's study led him to read the Bible. Paul is now dedicated to studying and living according to the Scriptures, and to developing his relationship with the Most High. It is Paul's prayer that people see the amazing health message of the Scriptures and getting to know and understand their Creator. It's his passion to teach everyone about the health and diet connection.

Paul is married to Andrea, and they have a daughter, Noa

Raquel. He and Andrea share the same passions for health, healing and the Scriptures.

RESOURCES

PAUL NISON
P.O. Box 16156
West Palm Beach, FL 33416
(917) 407-2270
E-mail: Paul@rawlife.com
www.Paulnison.com
This is the official website of author and raw food chef Paul Nison. See the website for Paul's teaching and lecture schedule.

RAW LIFE, INC.
P.O. Box 16156
West Palm Beach, FL 33416
toll-free (866) 729-7285, or 866-Raw-Paul
E-mail: Paul@rawlife.com
www.Rawlife.com
This is the best website for health books on all topics, including raw food diets and spiritual health. It also has a good selection of the highest quality raw food health snacks, foods, and supplements.

TORAH LIFE MINISTRIES
P.O. Box 16156
West Palm Beach, FL 33416
917-407-2270
E-mail: Paul@rawlife.com
www.Torahlifeministries.org
Torah Life Ministries, Inc., is a nonprofit ministry teaching the word of Yahweh (God), proclaiming the Good News of Yeshua (Jesus), and supporting the healing of all by revealing a more excellent way. It is our heart's desire to help fellow believers understand the important health message found in the Scriptures.
Visit Paul's blog page at www.Paulnison.com.
See many of Paul's videos now for free on www.RawLifeHealthShow.com or at www.Youtube.com.

HEALTH RESEARCH BOOKS
(888) 844-2386
www.healthresearchbooks.com
This is the world's largest publisher of rare and unusual health-related books. Nikki Jones and my friends at Health Research Books have reprinted Dr. Lewis's book Talks about People's Stomachs that is now available for purchase. You can order a copy through my website at www.Rawlife.com.

OTHER BOOKS BY PAUL NISON

THE RAW LIFE:
Becoming Natural in an Unnatural World

RAW KNOWLEDGE:
Enhance the Powers of Your Mind, Body, and Soul

HEALING INFLAMMATORY BOWEL DISEASE:
The Cause and Cure of Crohn's Disease
and Ulcerative Colitis

HEALTH ACCORDING TO THE SCRIPTURES:
Experience the Joy of Health
According to Our Creator

PAUL NISON'S RAW FOOD FORMULA FOR HEALTH:
A Modern Approach to Health Through Simplicity,
Variety, and Moderation

You can get these books and many of Paul's updated videos
and audios at www.Rawlife.com
or call toll-free (866) 729-7285, or 866-Raw-Paul.

BIBLIOGRAPHY

Bisci, Fred. *Your Healthy Journey: Discovering Your Body's Full Potential*, Staten Island, New York, Bisci Lifestyle Books, 2008.

Carrington, Hereward. *Death Deferred*, Pomeroy, Washington, Health Research Books, 1922.

Carrington, Hereward. *Fasting for Health and Long Life*, Pomeroy, Washington, Health Research Books, 1953.

Carrington, Hereward. *The Natural Food of Man*, Pomeroy, Washington, Health Research Books.

Cornaro, Luigi. *Discourses on the Sober Life*, Pomeroy, Washington, Health Research Books, 1560.

Ehret, Arnold. *The Mucusless Diet Healing System,* Dobbs Ferry, New York, Ehret Literature Publishing Company, 1953.

Ehret, Arnold. *Rational Fasting*, Dobbs Ferry, New York, Ehret Literature Publishing Company, 1926.

Ehret, Arnold. *The Cause and Cure of Disease,* Dobbs Ferry, New York, Ehret Literature Publishing Company, 2001.

Olver, Lynne. *The Food Timeline*, www.foodtimeline.org

Hotema, Hilton. *Man's Higher Consciousness,* Pomeroy, Washington: Health Research Books, 1962.

LaPallo, Bernando. *Age Less Live More*, self-published, 2008.

Lewis, Dio. *Talks about People's Stomachs,* Boston, Fields, Osgood and Company, 1870.

McMillan, Sherrie. *What Time is Dinner*, History Magazine, October/November 2001

Mr. Breakfast, *The Early Days of Breakfast Cereal,* www.Mrbreakfast.com

Peale, Norman Vincent. *Enthusiasm Makes the Difference*, Pawling, New York. Foundation for Christian Living.

White, Ellen. *Counsels on Diet and Foods*, The Ellen G. White Estate, Inc., 1976.

Zavasta, Tonya. *Quantum Eating: The Ultimate Elixir of Youth*, Cordova, Tennessee: BR Publishing, 2007.

"All diseases, without exception, even the hereditary, are caused — disregarding a few other hygienic causes — by biologically wrong, 'unnatural' food, and by each ounce of over-nourishment, only and exclusively." — **Professor Arnold Ehret**

INDEX

A

Adrenal fatigue *132, 135*

Air *225*

Arnold Ehret *71, 73, 120, 161, 167*

B

Bible *34, 57, 64, 100, 126*

Bisci, Fred *17, 18, 19, 21, 29, 34, 77, 86, 97, 121, 169*

blood *28, 29, 50, 64, 83, 95, 96, 121, 122, 134, 162, 165, 167, 168, 171, 208, 211, 212, 213, 216, 219*

bowel *27, 30, 165, 171, 208, 209, 213, 224. See* colon

C

cancer *28, 30, 92, 95, 132, 134, 208, 212, 227*

cleansing *30, 79, 94, 96, 101, 102, 106, 108, 109, 114, 123, 126, 161, 168, 169, 173, 204, 216*

colon *28, 30, 31, 32, 83, 84, 167, 173, 208. See* bowel

D

daylight *31, 37, 77, 81, 95, 99, 107, 108, 109, 126, 127, 129, 179, 187, 189, 199, 200, 203, 204, 220, 221*

daytime *44, 57, 84, 85, 108, 111, 112, 119, 127, 129, 141, 144, 145, 157, 186, 200, 220, 221*

detoxification *122, 162, 168*

digestion *27, 30, 31, 32, 33, 34, 35, 36, 45, 47, 58, 67, 69, 74, 77, 78, 79, 82, 83, 84, 91, 92, 93, 94, 96, 99, 100, 101, 103, 106, 107, 109, 110, 119, 122, 123, 124, 126, 143, 144, 145, 155, 161, 200, 202, 203, 208, 209, 210, 211, 213, 231, 242*

Dio Lewis *34, 53, 66, 92, 102, 116, 119, 141, 211, 227, 231*

E

Ehret, Arnold *21, 71, 73, 120, 161, 167*

F

fasting *33, 71, 72, 73, 77, 80, 120, 123, 168, 173*

Fred Bisci *17, 18, 19, 21, 29, 34, 77, 86, 97, 121, 169*

G

God *68, 78, 92, 94, 96, 185, 219, 225*

H

Hotema, Hilton *155*

L

Lewis, Dio *34, 53, 66, 92, 102, 116, 119, 141, 211, 227, 231*

light *46, 51, 53, 54, 61, 79, 91, 93, 94, 95, 97, 109, 110, 120, 127, 154, 197, 200, 225*

M

meals *28, 34, 35, 36, 41, 46, 47, 50, 51, 52, 53, 54, 55, 61, 62, 66, 69, 70, 73, 78, 79, 85, 86, 101, 104, 105, 106,*

107, 110, 115, 116, 117, 119, 120, 121, 122, 123, 124, 126, 127, 128, 129, 141, 142, 143, 147, 156, 157, 168, 172, 180, 193, 194, 197, 199, 200, 201, 202, 203, 204, 205, 209, 210, 221

moon *46, 94, 107, 124, 125, 196, 227, 233*

N

nighttime *40, 44, 49, 50, 51, 53, 54, 55, 66, 72, 78, 87, 94, 108, 119, 120, 126, 129, 132, 135, 141, 142, 143, 144, 145, 156, 157, 158, 164, 176, 178, 179, 181, 187, 188, 195, 201, 215, 220, 221, 225*

O

Overeating *30, 32, 69, 108, 164, 167*

R

raw food *31, 32, 33, 40, 41, 42, 87, 162, 181, 189, 210*

S

schedule *41, 45, 46, 51, 94, 98, 107, 108, 109, 110, 111, 112, 119, 120, 125, 126, 129, 130, 136, 137, 158, 159, 160, 178, 186, 187, 193, 194, 195, 196, 197, 202, 204, 217, 218, 219, 220, 227*

Scriptures *49, 111, 153, 225*

sleep *36, 40, 42, 43, 46, 47, 51, 52, 54, 69, 72, 74, 79, 80, 82, 87, 88, 92, 94, 99, 101, 102, 104, 105, 106, 107, 108, 109, 110, 111, 112, 113, 114, 119, 120, 124, 129, 133, 135, 137, 158, 160, 162, 164, 171, 177, 186, 194, 195, 196, 197, 200, 201, 203, 204, 208, 211, 212, 213, 225, 227, 229, 231*

sunshine *68, 93, 94, 223, 225*

W

White, Ellen *68, 155*